COMMON PATELLOFEMORAL PROBLEMS

EDITED BY
JOHN P. FULKERSON, MD
CLINICAL PROFESSOR AND SPORTS MEDICINE FELLOWSHIP DIRECTOR
DEPARTMENT OF ORTHOPAEDIC SURGERY
UNIVERSITY OF CONNECTICUT
ORTHOPAEDIC ASSOCIATES OF HARTFORD
FARMINGTON, CONNECTICUT

SERIES EDITOR
THOMAS R. JOHNSON, MD
ORTHOPAEDIC SURGEONS, PSC
BILLINGS, MONTANA

American Academy of Orthopaedic Surgeons

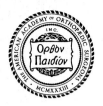

Common Patellofemoral Problems

Published by the
American Academy of Orthopaedic Surgeons
6300 North River Road
Rosemont, IL 60018
1-800-626-6726

The material presented in *Common Patellofemoral Problems* has been made available by the American Academy of Orthopaedic Surgeons for educational purposes only. This material is not intended to present the only, or necessarily best, methods or procedures for the medical situations discussed, but rather is intended to represent an approach, view, statement, or opinion of the author(s) or producer(s), which may be helpful to others who face similar situations.

Some drugs or medical devices demonstrated in Academy courses or described in Academy print or electronic publications have not been cleared by the Food and Drug Administration (FDA) or have been cleared for specific uses only. The FDA has stated that it is the responsibility of the physician to determine the FDA clearance status of each drug or device he or she wishes to use in clinical practice.

Furthermore, any statements about commercial products are solely the opinion(s) of the author(s) and do not represent an Academy endorsement or evaluation of these products. These statements may not be used in advertising or for any commercial purpose.

All rights reserved. No part of this publication may be reproduced, stored in a retrieval system, or transmitted, in any form, or by any means, electronic, mechanical, photocopying, recording, or otherwise, without prior written permission from the publisher.

Some of the authors or the departments with which they are affiliated have received something of value from a commercial or other party related directly or indirectly to the subject of their chapter.

First Edition
Copyright © 2005 by the
American Academy of
Orthopaedic Surgeons

ISBN 0-89203-349-5

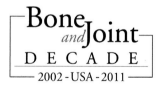

CONTRIBUTORS

Jack T. Andrish, MD
Staff Surgeon
Department of Orthopaedic Surgery
Cleveland Clinic Foundation
Cleveland, Ohio

Scott F. Dye, MD
Clinical Associate Professor of Orthopaedic Surgery
University of California, San Francisco
San Francisco, California

Jack Farr, MD
Director, Cartilage Restoration Center of Indiana
OrthoIndy
Indianapolis, Indiana

John P. Fulkerson, MD
Clinical Professor and Sports Medicine Fellowship Director
Department of Orthopaedic Surgery
University of Connecticut
Orthopaedic Associates of Hartford
Farmington, Connecticut

Ronald P. Grelsamer, MD
Department of Orthopaedic Surgery
The Hospital for Joint Diseases
New York, New York

Jeffrey L. Halbrecht, MD
Orthopaedic Surgeon
San Francisco, California

Michael A. Kelly, MD
Orthopaedic Surgery
Insall Scott Kelly Institute
New York, New York

Gwo-Chin Lee, MD
Insall Scott Kelly Institute
New York, New York

William R. Post, MD
Clinical Associate
West Virginia University
Department of Orthopaedics
Mountaineer Orthopaedic Specialists, LLC
Morgantown, West Virginia

Anthony A. Schepsis, MD
Professor of Orthopaedic Surgery
Director of Sports Medicine
Boston University Orthopaedic Surgical Associates
Boston University Medical Center
Boston, Massachusetts

Drew A. Stein, MD
Orthopaedic Surgeon
Maimonides Medical Center
Brooklyn, New York

Frederick J. Watson, MD
Tribury Orthopaedics, PC
Waterbury, Connecticut

CONTENTS

PREFACE VII

1 PATELLOFEMORAL PAIN WITHOUT MALALIGNMENT: A TISSUE HOMEOSTASIS PERSPECTIVE 1

2 PATELLOFEMORAL REALIGNMENT: PRINCIPLES AND GUIDELINES 11

3 ROTATIONAL MALALIGNMENT OF THE PATELLA 19

4 MILD PATELLAR INSTABILITY: ARTHROSCOPIC RECONSTRUCTION 29

5 ACUTE PATELLAR DISLOCATION 35

6 RECURRENT PATELLAR DISLOCATION 43

7 PATELLOFEMORAL ARTHRITIS WITH MALALIGNMENT . . 57

8 ISOLATED PATELLOFEMORAL ARTHRITIS WITHOUT MALALIGNMENT 73

9 PATELLOFEMORAL ARTICULAR CARTILAGE TREATMENT 85

INDEX 101

PREFACE

Patellofemoral pain and instability are more understandable now thanks to the research and contributions of many individuals over the past decade. The International Patellofemoral Study Group has encouraged collaborative efforts and consensus regarding patellofemoral pain and instability. In addition to the American authors in this AAOS treatise, the group in Lyon, France has contributed greatly to this understanding, particularly the work of David Dejour and Philippe Neyret, spearheaded by the earlier work of the great Henri Dejour. Other colleagues in Switzerland, Belgium, Italy, France, England, Brazil, Poland, Sweden, Norway, Germany, Spain, Australia, and Japan have provided important insights and collaboration.

While this little monograph cannot fully reflect all those who have contributed to understanding this topic, there is practical information here that should be helpful to orthopaedic surgeons, physicians, and physical therapists with interest in current surgical concepts regarding the management of patients with patellofemoral pain and instability.

Most important is to understand the nature of each patient's problem, treating nonsurgically until there is really no choice but to operate. Then, do only what is absolutely necessary and do it well. Patellofemoral problems do not lend themselves well to cookbook approaches, and nothing replaces a careful history and physical examination.

So the contents herein are only guidelines to help the careful clinician design an optimal plan for each patient based on a careful analysis of the patient's history and examination as well as selected imaging studies. Taking the time necessary to understand these disabled patients is rewarding for everyone involved.

John P. Fulkerson, MD
Editor

CHAPTER 1

PATELLOFEMORAL PAIN WITHOUT MALALIGNMENT: A TISSUE HOMEOSTASIS PERSPECTIVE

SCOTT F. DYE, MD

Patellofemoral pain is one of the most common, yet challenging conditions managed by orthopaedic surgeons. Despite extensive clinical experience and basic scientific research into patellofemoral pain, controversy remains regarding its etiology and appropriate treatment.[1] Most orthopaedic treatment for anterior knee pain assumes a purely structural and biomechanical etiology, namely, that chondromalacia and/or patellofemoral malalignment is the primary cause of the pain. This perspective, however, has often led to therapeutic approaches that actually worsen a patient's patellofemoral pain, including muscle strengthening exercises to correct maltracking and excessive use of surgical procedures such as lateral release, aggressive chondroplasties, and proximal and distal realignments.[1]

Recently, an alternative perspective on the etiology of patellofemoral pain has led to the development of a more logical and inherently safer therapeutic approach that is not based solely on structural and biomechanical factors.[1-4] This new paradigm de-emphasizes the importance of these structural and biomechanical factors and instead suggests that patellofemoral pain arises from the often transient loss of homeostasis in a variety of innervated patellofemoral tissues. This chapter discusses this new perspective and offers therapeutic recommendations for patients with patellofemoral pain without malalignment.

HISTORY

For decades, it has been assumed that chondromalacia of the patella is causally related to anterior knee pain; however, several studies have questioned this relationship.[5,6] For example, my patellae are totally pain free despite the documented presence of advanced chondromalacic damage. This damage was noted as an incidental finding during research surgery to delineate the neurosensory characteristics of the internal structures of the human knee without intra-articular anesthesia[7] (Fig. 1). Penetration of the unanesthetized synovium and fat pad tissues, however, produced severe pain (Fig. 2). Also, during earlier research to assess the intraosseous environment of the patella, transient increases of intraosseous pressure caused exquisite pain.[8]

TISSUE HOMEOSTASIS THEORY

These insights gained into the neurosensory characteristics of the patellofemoral joint, along with the results of other clinical studies, led to the development of the tissue

FIGURE 1

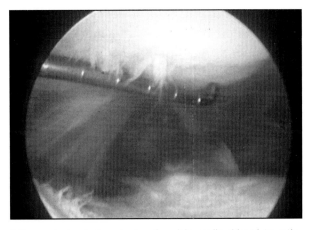

Arthroscopic view during palpation of my right patella without intra-articular anesthesia. No sensation was perceived, despite the presence of advanced chondromalacic damage.

FIGURE 2

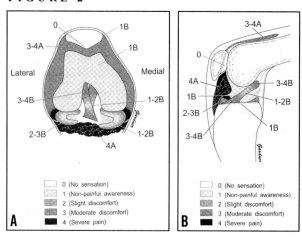

Neurosensory map of the intra-articular structures of the author's right knee as determined during research surgery. Coronal **(A)** and sagittal **(B)** views. A = accurate spatial localization of sensations. B = poorly localized sensations. *(Reproduced with permission from Dye SF, Vaupel GL, Dye CC: Conscious neuosensory mapping of the internal structures of the human knee. AM J Sports Med 1998;26:773-777.)*

homeostasis theory. Dye and associates[9] found that structural characteristics thought to be significant in the etiology of patellofemoral pain (eg, high Q angle, meniscus of sclerosis of the lateral facet of the patella) were not present at a statistically greater rate in symptomatic individuals than in age- and activity-matched asymptomatic control subjects. Further, the use of technetium Tc 99m methylene diphosphonate (MDP) scintigraphy revealed increased osseous metabolic activity of the patellae in many patients with anterior knee pain that reverted to normal (osseous homeostasis) with the resolution of symptoms following a successful nonsurgical treatment program.[8,10,11] Normal living structures, such as bone or ligaments, have the characteristic of tissue homeostasis as demonstrated by the constant maintenance of normal physiologic processes at the cellular and molecular levels, as well as the capability to restore normal physiologic processes following injury (ie, healing). The perception of pain both denotes the stimulation of peripheral nerves, alerting the central nervous system to injurious (or potentially injurious) conditions as part of an evolutionarily designed negative feedback loop, and connotes the loss of tissue homeostasis of innervated structures, such as patellar bone, or the irritation and inflammation of mechanically impinged peripatellar soft tissues.

The tissue homeostasis perspective appears to explain the often variable nature of patellofemoral pain from patient to patient more clearly than does the structural point of view. From this perspective, the variable nature of a patient's symptoms from day to day can be explained by possible loss of tissue homeostasis in the various innervated patellar and peripatellar tissues. Lancinating pain under conditions of patellofemoral loading could represent mechanical pinching of peripatellar synovium, a tissue that is documented to be well innervated.[4,7] These episodes of mechanical pinching often occur in knees without any evidence of patellofemoral malalignment. An effusion is also indicative of synovitis as one of the components of the mosaic of pathophysiologic processes that may account for patellofemoral pain.[3] The dull aching that many patients experience after certain loading activities is most likely the result of overload and subsequent irritation and inflammation of innervated tissues. The absence of pain reflects loading that is nonirritating to those same tissues. The "movie theater sign," or the experience of dull aching with prolonged knee flexion, is most likely the result of transient increases in intraosseous pressure caused by slight venous outflow obstruction that resolves rapidly with extension or ambulation. Variables not directly related to patellofemoral loading, such as anterior knee pain secondary to changes of barometric pressure, may seem to be confounding, but this phenomenon may be attributed to barosensitivity of the intraosseous environment, as well as sensitized peripatellar tissues. Further, Fulkerson and associates,[12] Biedert and associates,[13,14] and Sanchis-Alfonso and associates[15,16] demonstrated that the presence of painful neuromata in the retinaculae and other peripatellar tissues may also play a role in the genesis of patellofemoral symptoms. These painful neuromas represent a direct neuropathophysiologic source of nociception. Small neuromata cannot be imaged by any current technology, including MRI, and are often diagnosed clinically by tenderness to palpation, a positive Tinel's sign, and with histologic studies following surgical excision. Wojtys and associates[17] demonstrated that substance-P, a neuroactive peptide within the peripatellar soft tissues, can also be a part of the pathophysiologic process, ultimately resulting in the perception of anterior knee pain. The pathophysiologic factors that are likely to induce patellofemoral pain are listed in Table 1.[4]

FUNCTION OF THE KNEE

The knee can be thought of as a biologic transmission system, the purpose of which is to accept, redirect, and dissipate a range of biomechanical loads.[18] The patellofemoral joint can be visualized as a large slide bearing within this living, self-maintaining, self-repairing transmission system. Ligaments can be seen as sensate adaptive linkages, and the menisci viewed as mobile, sensate bearings. In this analogy, the muscles function as living cellular engines that provide motive forces across the knee (transmission) in concentric contraction and absorb and dissipate shock loads in eccentric contraction. The importance of eccentric muscle contraction is emphasized by Winter,[19] who demonstrated that the muscles about the knee actually absorb more than three times the energy that is generated in motive forces.

The functional capacity of a joint to safely and painlessly accept and transfer a range of loads, and yet maintain tissue homeostasis, is represented by a load/frequency distribution termed the envelope of function or the envelope of load acceptance[18] (Fig. 3, A). If too little load is placed across a joint for an extended period of time (eg, prolonged bed rest), loss of tissue homeostasis may result, manifested by muscle atrophy and disuse osteopenia. This region of diminished load is termed the zone of subphysiologic underload (Fig. 3, B). If excessive loads—

beyond the range of acceptable physiologic limits but insufficient to cause macrostructural damage—are placed across a joint, loss of tissue homeostasis can ensue (eg, a stress fracture of the tibia in a long-distance runner). This loss is manifested in bone by a positive technetium Tc 99m bone scan before radiographic changes are evident. This region of excessive loading is termed the zone of supraphysiologic overload. If sufficiently great loads are placed across a joint or musculoskeletal system, then overt macrostructural damage can occur (eg, a fracture of bone or rupture of a ligament). The region of excessive loading resulting in overt structural damage is termed the zone of structural failure.

In my opinion, the most common loss of tissue homeostasis important in the origin of patellofemoral pain is in the patient with normal patellofemoral alignment who sustains loading into the region of supraphysiologic overload through either a single event or with repetitive loading (Fig. 3, C). The tissues of the patellofemoral joint sustain the highest loading of any joint and often function at or near the limits of biologic load acceptance and transference capacity. Thus, these are often the first knee tissues to be loaded to the point of supraphysiologic failure, leading to symptomatic loss of tissue homeostasis that is manifested by patellofemoral pain. The envelope of function frequently diminishes after an injury to a level where many activities of daily living that were previously well tolerated may become symptomatic (out of the envelope of function) and result in prolonged symptoms (Fig. 3, D). Decreasing the loading across a symptomatic joint to within the newly diminished envelope of function allows normal tissue healing processes to proceed to homeostasis most rapidly without recurrent subversion (Fig. 3, E). This restriction of loading to a pain-free level is the clear purpose of the neurologic sensors that act as part of a negative feedback loop, and it also corresponds to the patient's common sense. Recurrent painful loading out of the envelope, such as excessive stair climbing or squatting, subverts the normal healing processes and is the hallmark of chronic patellofemoral pain in many patients.

The fundamental goal of treating patients with patellofemoral pain is restoration of painless knee function. The tissue homeostasis perspective is inherently empiric and thus fundamentally safer than many current therapeutic approaches that are based solely on correction of structural and biomechanical factors thought to be of causal significance.[20] These structurally and biome-

---

TABLE 1

Factors Inducing Patellofemoral Nociceptive Output

Mechanical environment
    Direct patellofemoral trauma
    Excessive intrinsic compressive and tensile forces
        Normal alignment
        Malalignment (load shifting)
    Impingement of intra-articular structures
    Increased intraosseous pressure
    Barometric pressure changes
Chemical environment
    Presence of cytokines
    Altered pH of damaged tissues
Localized peripheral neuropathy
    Painful neuroma
Nonpatellofemoral sources
    Referred pain (such as hip arthrosis)
    Phantom limb pain in transfemoral amputees

(Reproduced with permission from Dye SF, Vaupel GL, Dye CC: Conscious neurosensory mapping of the internal structures of the human knee without intra-articular anesthesia. Am J Sports Med 1998;26:773-777.)

FIGURE 3

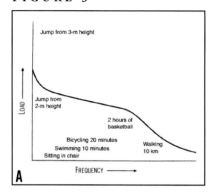
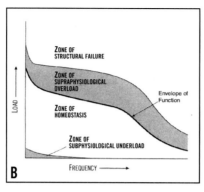
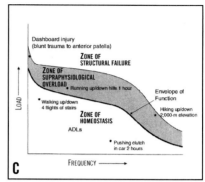
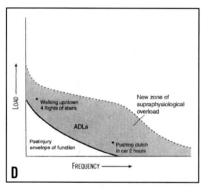
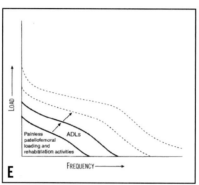

A, Hypothetical graph representing the envelope of function for an athletically active young adult. The graph represents loads associated with different activities. All of the loading examples, except a jump from a 3-m height, are within the envelope for this particular knee. The shape of the envelope of function represented here is an idealized theoretical model. The actual loads transmitted across an individual knee under these different conditions are variable and are the result of multiple complex factors, including the dynamic center of gravity, the rate of load application, and the angles of flexion and rotation. The limits of the envelope of function for the joint of an actual patient are probably more complex. **B,** Hypothetical graph showing the four zones of loading across a joint. The area within the envelope of function is the zone of homeostasis. In the zone of supraphysiologic overload, loading is greater than that within the envelope of function but is insufficient to cause macrostructural damage. The region of loading that is great enough to cause macrostructural damage is the zone of structural failure. The region of decreased loading over time resulting in a loss of tissue homeostasis is the zone of subphysiologic underload. **C,** Supraphysiologic loads outside the envelope: a dashboard injury, running up and down hills for 1 hour, and hiking up and down a 2,000-m elevation. **D,** Diminished envelope of function after supraphysiologic patellofemoral loading showing that ADLs and activities such as climbing four flights of stairs and pushing a clutch in a vehicle for 2 hours have become suprisiologic loads, leading to recurrent loss of tissue homeostasis and continuance of peripatellar symptoms. **E,** Incremental expansion of the diminished envelope of function by restricting patellofemoral loading to within the envelope. *(Reproduced with permission from Dye SF, Staubli HU, Biedert R: The mosaic of pathophysiology causing patellofemoral pain.* Oper Tech Sports Med *1999;7:46-54.)*

chanically oriented approaches often result in the worsening of patellofemoral symptoms. For example, an aggressive physical therapy program that solely emphasizes vastus medialis obliquus strengthening to correct maltracking by extension of the knee against resistance often results in increased anterior knee pain. Such a narrow emphasis on muscle strengthening at the expense of increased patellofemoral symptoms is inherently illogical. Further, many currently accepted surgical approaches for patients with patellofemoral pain such as lateral release, aggressive chondroplasties for findings of chondromalacia, and major proximal and/or distal realignment surgery are based solely on structural and biomechanical characteristics and may inadvertently result in worsen-ing of symptoms.[20] In my experience, the worst patellofemoral pain and dysfunction occur in patients who have had multiple surgical procedures for symptoms that initially were only mild or intermittent patellofemoral discomfort.

HISTORY AND PHYSICAL EXAMINATION

Before beginning treatment, the most specific diagnosis possible should be established. Assessment should concentrate on the history and physical examination, rather than imaging studies. A thorough history will often elicit an underlying supraphysiologic loading event or series of events that preceded the onset of symptoms. It is not unusual, however, for patients to be unable to identify a specific occurrence of causal significance. Patients may simply report that certain activities of daily living (ADLs) associated with high patellofemoral loading, such as stair climbing, squatting, kneeling, prolonged sitting, or arising from chairs, elicit symptoms. Patellofemoral instability, such as a patellar dislocation, should be excluded as a cause of symptoms. The treatment of patellofemoral instability is not within the scope of this chapter.

The clinical examination should localize the pain and tenderness and identify which loading activities contribute significantly to the anterior knee pain. Specific sites of tenderness often lead to specific diagnoses, such as retinacular strain, synovitis, or tendinitis. Have the patient reproduce, if possible, the activities that induce patellofemoral pain. For example, the knee can be assessed under load by having the patient step up and down off a footstool. The exact activities associated with the initiation and persistence of patellofemoral symptoms should be identified so that they can be rigorously restricted. Such supraphysiologic pain-inducing activities are, by definition, outside the individual's envelope of function. Observe the muscle bulk, patellar tracking characteristics, and overall alignment of the limb. Determine if nonpatellofemoral sources, such as tight hamstrings or referred pain from arthritis of the hip or saphenous nerve irritation, contribute to the symptoms.

IMAGING

Standard screening radiographs of both knees, including Merchant or Laurin views, should be obtained to rule out overt structural causes of pain, such as fractures or loose bodies.[21,22] Minor degrees of tilting and subluxation of the patella relative to the femoral trochlea on axial radiographs, in my opinion, reveal little regarding the cause of anterior knee pain, and care should be taken to not overinterpret such findings.[9] Stäubli and associates[23] demonstrated that the articular cartilage morphology often does not match the osseous morphology. Patellar articular cartilage that appears tilted on radiographs may in fact mate well with the trochlear articular cartilage. In such cases, surgery that results in the absence of tilt on postoperative radiographs may inadvertently create an iatrogenic malalignment.

Dye and associates[9] documented that mild degrees of patellar tilt and subluxation did not correlate well with the presence or absence of anterior knee pain. Further, MRI is poor at identifying which of the patellofemoral tissues is the source of pain. Even identifiable structural damage to articular cartilage does not necessarily contribute to anterior knee symptoms, as previously noted. Therefore, even with findings of extensive chondromalacic damage of patellar articular cartilage, the patient may be totally asymptomatic.[7] Coincidentally, a technetium Tc 99m-MDP bone scan of my knees was obtained at the time of the research surgery and the findings were normal. In combination, these findings exemplify the principle that the presence of tissue homeostasis is often more important relative to the absence of symptoms than the documented presence of structural damage.[11] Therefore, extreme caution should be taken when ascribing causality of patellofemoral pain to structural findings such as chondromalacia on MRI.

A careful examination of MRI scans of the patellofemoral joint often reveals low-grade effusions associated with symptomatic peripatellar synovitis, a finding that often goes unreported by radiologists because of their focus on evaluating the structural characteristics of joints. Therefore, it is important for the treating orthopaedic surgeon to meticulously examine these images directly. Technetium Tc 99m bone scans, which manifest loss of osseous homeostasis, often correlate well with patellar pain and its resolution.[8,10,11]

TREATMENT

Nonsurgical

The treatment of patients with patellofemoral pain without malalignment from a tissue homeostasis perspective is a logical, empirically based program that aims to expand the envelope of function for a given patient's knee to its maximum as safely and predictably as possible. The goal is to help the patient create an internal biologic environment in the symptomatic joint that is most conducive to restoration of tissue homeostasis (healing) with the associated resolution of pain. Each patient's condition, which is a function of a mosaic of possible pathophysiologic processes, and healing potential are unique; therefore, treatment should be individualized. In my experience, most patients with patellofemoral pain have a positive response to the application of three basic principles: (1) correcting the pathokinematics by temporarily but scrupulously adhering to load restriction within the patient's reduced envelope of function; (2) an anti-inflammatory treatment program; and (3) rehabilitation.

Load Restriction

Loads across the symptomatic patellofemoral joint must be diminished to the point where they are no longer causing further tissue damage or irritation. In other words, the patient must decrease the loading across the symptomatic joint to within the diminished envelope of function, or to a range of loading that is currently clinically painless. The patient must be made aware that continuing painful loading activities will hinder normal tissue healing processes. Analogies can be helpful in explaining these concepts to patients. For example, one of the most important of the pathophysiologic processes associated with anterior knee pain is patellofemoral synovitis. This condition can be likened to repeatedly biting the inside of a swollen cheek, in which case the painful loss of homeostasis represented by the irritated tissues can persist indefinitely. Often the activities that are associated with persistent patellofemoral pain are readily identifiable and controllable. Simple modifications of ADLs such as limiting excessive stair climbing, squatting, kneeling, and other pain-inducing activities that are out of the patient's envelope of function; changing the manner in which one sits in and arises from a chair; and sitting in a higher chair to keep the knee in a more extended position are often sufficient to achieve a painless range of patellofemoral loading. For women, in particular, the temporary use of an elevated toilet seat can be beneficial. When resting, patients should keep the knee in a more extended position to prevent the deep aching associated with the "movie theater sign."

Anti-inflammatory Treatment

Most anterior knee pain, in my experience, is at least partially the result of an inflammatory process that is most often reflected in the production of cytokine enzymes within irritated synovial tissues and other innervated tissues.[3,4] Any of these inflamed tissues may respond well to intermittent tissue cooling and oral nonsteroidal anti-inflammatory drugs of the surgeon's choice. Patients fre-

quently report improvement of patellofemoral pain with a repetitive tissue cooling program of icing for 15 to 20 minutes two to three times a day, particularly after performing activities that aggravate the patellofemoral joint. The symptomatic benefit of tissue cooling most likely reflects both a temporary decrease in swelling of inflamed peripatellar tissues and decreased metabolic activity that results in a transient decrease in cytokine production within the inflamed innervated tissues. The patient should be cautioned against overcooling the knee and causing a new iatrogenic hypothermal injury.[2]

Rehabilitation

Rehabilitation that includes a combination of painless muscle strengthening, stretching, and patellofemoral taping often is beneficial in creating an internal biomechanical environment that encourages maximal tissue healing. Some degree of muscle atrophy is not uncommon in patients with patellofemoral pain. Atrophy is often interpreted as a primary etiologic fac-tor, but it may actually be secondary to disuse. Muscle strengthening, including the vastus medialis obliquus, is considered beneficial in most patients, but such strengthening exercises must be performed in a painless manner–that is, within the envelope of function for that individ-ual patient. For example, strengthening exercises for the quadriceps musculature that includes painful extension of the knee against resistance may aggravate already sensitive and inflamed peripatellar tissues. Exercises that are beneficial for the muscles may be injurious for the knee joint itself. Passive stretching of tight structures, such as the hamstrings and retinacula, is helpful and should be performed in a slow, measured manner so as to avoid new tissue injury. The absence of pain is the best indicator that the involved structures are not being reinjured.

McConnell patellar taping may result in noticeable pain reduction.[24] In my opinion, the often dramatic improvement of patellofemoral discomfort possible with this technique reflects a decrease in mechanical irritation of peripatellar tissue (not unlike using a finger to pull the swollen cheek tissue away from the teeth) rather than a correction of patellofemoral malalignment. Taping may also increase the beneficial proprioceptive characteristics of the patellofemoral joint. Because of skin irritation, McConnell taping is best used temporarily to protect the symptomatic joint while tissue homeostasis and healing occurs rather than long term. Other external devices, such as braces that place a medially directed vector onto the patella, can simulate McConnell taping. If these external techniques help reduce pain, they should be used; if symptoms are made worse, they should be discontinued. The use of nonrigid orthotics also can benefit many patients.

A treatment program must be individualized and empiric, meaning that it should be designed to help the patient find his or her specific envelope of function, and should include anti-inflammatory therapy and exercise programs that most reliably result in pain reduction. Each patient's program will be unique and should be chosen from inherently safe treatment choices. Once the painful symptoms have improved, the patient may gradually and incrementally increase patellofemoral loading activities. Using technetium Tc 99m scintigraphy, Dye and associates[9] demonstrated that resolution of patellofemoral pain and restoration of osseous homeostasis occurs over a 6- to 9-month period of nonsurgical treatment; however, many patients experience resolution of their symptoms much sooner. Adherence to the principles of this program offers the best chance of success. The first day the patient experiences the absence of pain does not mean that the envelope of function has been fully restored but that healing is occurring. Therefore, the patient should continue with a successful treatment approach rather than return to high loading activities immediately.

A tissue homeostasis approach to patellofemoral pain is inherently safe because any treatment factor that results in increased symptoms of patellofemoral pain is stopped immediately. When in doubt, the patient should be encouraged to decrease loading and go to the safe region of the envelope of function. No one program or approach will work for all patients because the underlying pathophysiology and tissue healing characteristics are unique to each patient.

Surgical

If symptoms persist despite a careful nonsurgical approach, surgery can then be considered as part of a tissue homeostasis approach to patellofemoral pain. However, surgical decisions must be approached rationally and cautiously with therapeutic approaches that take into account the special characteristics of this anatomic region of the knee. As previously noted, the worst patellofemoral pain and dysfunction I have witnessed were in patients who had only mild and intermittent symptoms and subsequently underwent multiple surgical procedures in an attempt to correct a supposed chondromalacia or malalignment etiology. Surgery performed from a tissue homeostasis perspective must be logically aimed at those aspects of the pathophysiology determined to be respon-

sible for the genesis of anterior knee pain and also most amenable to surgical correction. Not all factors that induce anterior knee pain are surgically correctable; therefore, improvement, rather than complete restoration of painless function after surgery, is most common. Surgical procedures must be done in a conservative manner that respects the special biologic and biomechanical nature of the patellofemoral joint so as not to create additional permanent injury to the joint.

In my experience, most patients with chronic peripatellar pain that fails to resolve with nonsurgical treatment

FIGURE 4

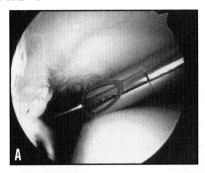

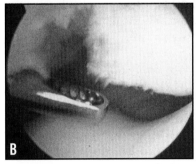

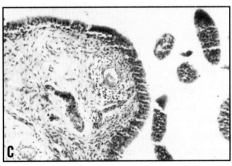

Arthroscopic peripatellar synovectomy. **A,** Peripatellar synovitis and chondromalacia. **B,** Peripatellar synovectomy and gentle chondroplasty. **C,** Histologic findings of tissue removed arthroscopically showing thickening and lymphocyte infiltration typical of chronic inflamed peripatellar synovitis (Hematoxylin & Eosin; original magnification, × 250).

will demonstrate peripatellar synovitis as a substantial aspect of their condition.[1,3,4] A carefully performed arthroscopic peripatellar synovectomy can be helpful (Fig. 4). The surgical removal of swollen peripatellar synovium can often be performed without technical difficulty. The challenge lies in providing postoperative management that results in a maximally functional envelope. Inflamed synovium must be cleared so that the inferior articular cartilage surface of the patella can be visualized. Following the peripatellar synovectomy, it is imperative that a hemarthrosis be avoided through meticulous intraoperative hemostasis and the use of a drain. A ⅛-in-diameter drain attached to a low-level vacuum source is suggested for a few hours following surgery, or on occasion, overnight, depending on the output. In addition, a subsynovial injection of 1% lidocaine and 1/100,000 epinephrine (approximately 40 mL) is recommended before the end of surgery, and 50 mL of 0.25% marcaine with 1/200,000 epinephrine and 10 mg of morphine should be injected sterilely into the knee through a drain tubing, which is then clamped for a period of up to 1 hour. After instillation of the marcaine mixture, a compressive dressing is applied, including the use of a thigh-high compression stocking. The dressing is removed the first postoperative day. Patients are then encouraged to remain at a low level of activity for several days after surgery to allow repopulation of new synovial cells. This temporary restriction of loading after surgery is described to patients as similar to letting a soufflé set without banging the oven door. It is also helpful to ice the knee 5 to 6 times a day for 15 or 20 minutes to decrease swelling and cytokine production. Pain-free straight leg raising and weight bearing as tolerated are recommended, along with the initiation of a painless postoperative rehabilitation program the week after surgery.

Chondroplasty can be beneficial to stabilize a region of chondral damage; however, it should be performed gently. Aggressive drilling, mosaicplasties, or cartilage transplantation techniques in the patellofemoral joint are inherently more traumatic and have yet to be proved safe and effective in long-term follow-up. The biomechanical environment in this region appears to be just too severe for long-term success with most current cartilage replacement techniques. Future research, however, should lead to the development of improved techniques. In addition, the removal of loose bodies can be beneficial. A lateral release should be performed solely in the setting of a documented tight lateral retinaculum, as described by

Fulkerson and associates.[12] Despite seeing many patients with patellofemoral pain, I rarely perform more than one or two lateral releases per year. Also, the use of lateral release within the International Patellofemoral Study Group has dramatically decreased within the past decade, as it has been recognized that this operation is not a panacea and has its own inherently dangerous characteristics.

Major proximal and distal realignment procedures for patellofemoral pain are inherently more dangerous because they often involve extensive tissue dissection and/or osteotomy of bone. The long-term results of these procedures are fundamentally unpredictable, despite how well the patellofemoral joint appears to be functioning at surgery. This unpredictability is attributed to factors beyond the surgeon's control, including the development of differential postoperative muscular atrophy and possible alteration of cerebellar sequencing of motor unit firing, resulting in altered patellofemoral kinematics. In most cases, major surgery should be contemplated only for demonstrated recurrent symptomatic patellofemoral instability or for established patellofemoral arthrosis. The use of anterior medial transfer of the tibial tubercle can be helpful in such cases. These procedures, however, are not without risk, and early, as well as late tibial stress fractures have been reported.[25,26] Other procedures that involve greater surgical perturbation, such as patellectomy and unicompartmental arthroplasty, should also be considered only in the face of severe established patellofemoral arthrosis.

CONCLUSIONS

The human body's ability to restore tissue homeostasis (healing) of injured highly loaded tissues involved in the genesis of patellofemoral pain is the result of billions of years of molecular and cellular evolutionary refinements. Therefore, treatment is most likely to be successful if it respects the special biologic and biomechanical nature of the patellofemoral joint, as in an empiric nonsurgical treatment program that is designed to maximize healing and minimize symptoms as predictably and safely as possible. If this approach fails, a careful, logical surgical approach may be considered.

REFERENCES

1. Dye SF: Patellofemoral pain current concepts: An overview. *Sports Med Arth Rev* 2001;9:264-272.

2. Dye SF: Therapeutic implications of a tissue homeostasis approach to patellofemoral pain. *Sports Med Arth Rev* 2001; 9:306-311.

3. Dye SF, Stäubli HU, Beidert RM, Vaupel GL: The mosaic of pathophysiology causing patellofemoral pain: Therapeutic implications. *Oper Tech Sports* 1999;7:46-54.

4. Dye SF, Vaupel GL: The pathophysiology of patellofemoral pain. *Sports Med Arth Rev* 1994;2:203-210.

5. DeHaven KE, Collins HR: Diagnosis of internal derangements of the knee: The role of arthroscopy. *J Bone Joint Surg Am* 1975;57:802-810.

6. McGinty JB, McCarthy JC: Endoscopic lateral retinacular release: A preliminary report. *Clin Orthop* 1981;158:120.

7. Dye SF, Vaupel GL, Dye CC: Conscious neurosensory mapping of the internal structures of the human knee without intra-articular anesthesia. *Am J Sports Med* 1998; 26:773-777.

8. Dye SF, Chew MH: The use of scintigraphy to detect increased osseous metabolic activity about the knee. *J Bone Joint Surg Am* 1993;75:1388-1406.

9. Dye SF, Boll DH, Dunigan PE, et al: An analysis of objective measurements including radionuclide imaging in young patients with patellofemoral pain. *Am J Sports Med* 1985;13:432.

10. Dye SF, Boll DA: Radionuclide imaging of the patellofemoral joint in young adults with anterior knee pain. *Orthop Clin North Am* 1986;17:249-262.

11. Dye SF, Peartree PK: Sequential radionuclide imaging of the patellofemoral joint in symptomatic young adults. *Am J Sports Med* 1989;17:727.

12. Fulkerson JP, Tennant R, Jaivin JS, et al: Histologic evidence of retinacular nerve injury associated with patellofemoral malalignment. *Clin Orthop* 1985;197:196-205.

13. Biedert RM, Stauffer E, Friederich NF: Occurrence of free nerve endings in the soft tissue of the knee joint: A histological investigation. *Am J Sports Med* 1992;20:430-433.

14. Biedert RM, Kernan V: Neurosensory characteristics of the patellofemoral joint: What is the genesis of patellofemoral pain? *Sports Med Arth Rev* 2001;9:295-300.

15. Sanchis-Alfonso V, Rosello-Sastre E, Monteagudo-Castro C, Esquerdo J: Quantitative analysis of nerve changes in the lateral retinaculum in patients with isolated symptomatic patellofemoral malalignment. *Am J Sports Med* 1998; 26:703-709.

16. Sanchis-Alfonso V, Rosello-Sastre E: Immunohistochemical analysis for neural markers of the lateral retinaculum in patients with isolated symptomatic patellofemoral malalignment: A neuroanatomical basis for anterior knee pain in the active young patient. *Am J Sports Med* 2000; 28:725-731.

17. Wojtys EM, Beaman DN, Guner RA, Janda D: Innervation of the human knee joint by substance-P fibers. *Arthroscopy* 1990;6:254-263.

18. Dye SF: The knee as a biologic transmission with an envelope of function. *Clin Orthop* 1996;325:10-18.

19. Winter DA: Energy generation and absorption at the ankle and knee during fast, natural, and slow cadences. *Clin Orthop* 1983;175:147-154.

20. Hillsgrove DC, Paulos LE: Complications of patellofemoral surgery, in *The Patella*. Berlin, Germany, Springer-Verlag, 1995, pp 277-290.

21. Merchant AC, Mercer RL, Jacobsen RH, et al: Roentgenographic analysis of patellofemoral congruence. *J Bone Joint Surg Am* 1974;56:1391-1396.

22. Laurin CA, Dussault R, Leveque HP: The tangential x-ray investigation of the patellofemoral joint: X-ray technique, diagnostic criteria and their interpretation. *Clin Orthop* 1979;144:16-26.

23. Stäubli HU, Durrenmatt U, Porcellini B, Rauschning W: Anatomy and surface geometry of the patellofemoral joint in the axial plane. *J Bone Joint Surg Br* 1999;81:452-458.

24. Grelsamer RP, McConnell J: *The Patella: A Team Approach.* Gaithersburg, MD, Aspen Publishers, 1998.

25. Fulkerson JP: Fracture of the proximal tibia after Fulkerson anterior medial tibial tubercle transfer: A report of four cases. *Am J Sports Med* 1999;27:265.

26. Eager MR, Bader DA, Kelly JD, Moyer RA: Delayed fracture of the tibia following medialization, osteotomy of the tibial tubercle: A report of five cases. *Am J Sports Med* 2004;22:1041-1048.

PATELLOFEMORAL REALIGNMENT: PRINCIPLES AND GUIDELINES

JOHN P. FULKERSON, MD

Improved understanding of the anatomy of the anterior knee has spurred a renewed interest in methods of reconstructing the unstable or malaligned extensor mechanism of the knee. Articular cartilage resurfacing options give new hope to patients with articular damage related to patellar instability, and anteromedial tibial tubercle transfer allows simultaneous realignment and unloading of the patella. Successful realignment or stabilization of the knee extensor mechanism is possible in most patients by adhering to rigorous principles and cautious guidelines. Each patient is different, however, so the surgeon must consider carefully all structural, functional, articular, and psychological factors.

THE PROBLEM

Management of anterior knee instability is a complicated issue, and no single option is best for all patients. The goal is to find the most accurate, least invasive method of treatment, and this involves sorting through the many structural and functional factors leading to extensor mechanism malalignment and dysfunction.[1] Initially, nonsurgical options should be rigorously pursued.

Laxity or imbalance of the extensor mechanism causes pain in various ways, such as by aberrant articular loading, small nerve injury in the retinaculum, chronic strain (resulting in pain similar to what occurs in patients with multidirectional shoulder instability), and synovial irritation. Lower extremity balance and timing are important in patients with patellofemoral instability.[2,3] Weak hip external rotators and abductors in women affect lower limb control (Fig. 1). These factors, which are known to contribute to an increased risk of anterior cruciate ligament rupture in women,[2] pertain to patellofemoral instability

and pain as well. When the hip is weak, obligate internal rotation of the lower extremity may functionally induce or aggravate patellar malalignment and result in symptoms of either patellar instability or pain.

FIGURE 1

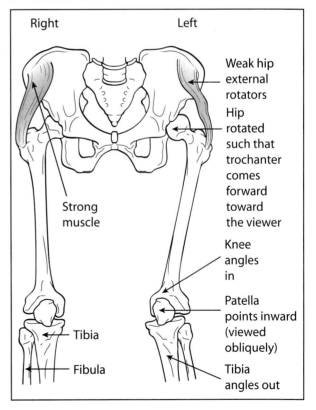

Effect of weak hip external rotators on lower limb and extensor mechanism alignment.

NONSURGICAL TREATMENT

Patients who have lower extremity imbalance with anterior knee pain or instability must undergo meticulous rehabilitation that includes strengthening and balancing of the entire lower body,[4,5] patellar taping,[6] bracing with one of the current improved braces (my preference is the Donjoy Ortho TruPull brace, Vista, CA), mobilization of tight structures, and anti-inflammatory drugs for pain. Nonsurgical treatment should also include plyometric strengthening, proprioceptive training, and traditional eccentric and concentric exercises. Closed-chain exercises may offer some advantages.[7] Despite optimal nonsurgical treatment, many patients continue to have disabling instability or pain emanating from the extensor mechanism. When faced with this situation, the surgeon must decide which surgical procedure to use.

IDENTIFYING THE CAUSE OF PAIN

The cause of patellofemoral pain can be elusive. Each of the possibilities listed in Table 1 must be considered.

PATIENT SELECTION

To ensure optimal surgical outcome, the surgeon must make certain that the patient is a good candidate for surgery both psychologically and physically. A patient must have reasonable motivation and exhibit psychological stability to gain benefit from surgery. Psychological screening may be helpful in selected patients. If there are questions about psychological status, counseling may be advisable. Some patients need antidepressant medication, and others may require treatment for complex regional pain syndrome, which must be resolved before undertaking patellofemoral reconstruction.

Patients who are smokers or obese and patients with diabetes mellitus are considered at higher risk for complications after patellofemoral surgery. Patients should be counseled appropriately in smoking cessation, weight loss, treatment of diabetes mellitus, establishing a normal nutritional status, and controlling depression with medication if necessary.

SURGICAL TREATMENT

The choice of surgical treatment depends on the source of the patellofemoral pain as well as other factors. Identifying the source(s) of pain requires a meticulous clinical examination. The goal is to avoid unnecessary patellar release or realignment and make treatment as specific as possible. The following considerations can help guide the choice of surgical treatment.

Soft-Tissue Sources of Pain

The peripatellar retinaculum is often an important source of pain and should be given careful consideration[8-11] (Fig. 2). Any soft-tissue source of pain should be treated directly either by injection or release. Some patients gain great benefit with extremely limited surgical intervention or injection if the surgeon identifies a specific retinacular or

---

TABLE 1

Causes of Patellofemoral Pain

True subchondral pain related to overload

Synovitis or fat pad pain

Retinacular pain related to imbalance and overload on the retinaculum

Retinacular pain related to a specific neuroma or enthesopathy

Peripatellar pain related to instability (analogous to multidirectional instability of the shoulder)

Referred pain from the quadriceps, hip, or back

Patellar or quadriceps tendinitis

Complex regional pain syndrome

FIGURE 2

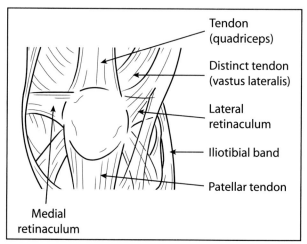

The peripatellar retinaculum is richly innervated and may be a primary source of pain.

soft-tissue source of pain such as symptomatic pathologic plicae, indurated or resistant patellar tendinitis, neuroma, painful scar, suture pain, retinacular pain, quadriceps muscle pain (including skeletal muscle hemangioma), or localized intra-articular synovitis. Realignment procedures and nonspecific surgical procedures are unnecessary in these patients.

Patellar Tilt

When there is radiographic and clinical evidence of patellar tilt, lateral retinacular release is frequently helpful provided that no load is placed on a lesion.[12,13] Lateral release may provide good results when there is lateral facet articular softening related to chronic tilt; however, lateral release will not consistently or reliably correct subluxation (Fig. 3).

Articular Lesions

Many patients with chronic patellofemoral pain have symptomatic articular lesions. These lesions tend to be distal/central or lateral and related to abnormal shear stress and overload in the chronically lateralized patella. A dislocation may result in a large medial facet lesion, which may or may not be symptomatic. Any selected procedure must avoid overloading the lesion and, in some cases, a cartilage resurfacing procedure is performed in conjunction with realignment to minimize or eliminate load on the lesion. Reproducible clinical criteria should

FIGURE 3

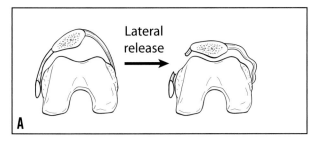

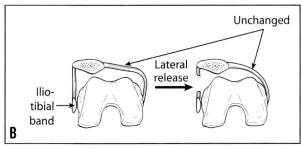

Lateral retinacular release relieves tilt (**A**) but not subluxation (**B**).

be used to establish that the articular lesion is the source of pain because some lesions may be incidental and not a specific cause of pain.

Arthroscopic or Mini-Open Medial Imbrication

Arthroscopic proximal medial imbrication can be helpful following lateral release when there is stretch of the medial retinaculum and medial patellofemoral ligament (MPFL) related to subluxation or dislocation of the patella. No long-term results are available to show that arthroscopic medial imbrication provides permanent stability enhancement. The procedure has limited usefulness, and mini-open medial imbrication is a reasonable alternative. Patients should be advised that this may be a temporizing procedure. Arthroscopic or mini-open medial imbrication should include specific suturing or tensioning of the MPFL, particularly if there has been a dislocation and disruption with subsequent scar formation in that region. I believe it is important to visualize and palpate the region of the MPFL to ensure the presence and proper orientation of tissue to imbricate, and therefore prefer the mini-open approach in most cases. Advancement of the vastus medialis obliquus (VMO) also tightens the remnant of MPFL (which inserts on the underside of the VMO), but ligamentous tissue in the proper orientation (inserting at the adductor tubercle/medial epicondyle region) must be present. I prefer to use cruciate stitches to gather tissue and minimize slippage through the MPFL fibers. Arthroscopic imbrication may reduce laxity of the patellofemoral joint as a cause of pain, analogous to reducing shoulder instability in multidirectional shoulder instability. In this way, arthroscopic imbrication may reduce or eliminate microinstability that is causing chronic capsular strain and pain. Arthroscopic imbrication may be best used to temporize, with hope of long-term success in patients with less malalignment, normal trochlea, and definable tissue to imbricate. I am currently partial to mini-open MPFL advancement, with the VMO, through a 3-cm incision. I also use arthroscopic imbrication selectively.

Reconstruction of the Medial Patellofemoral Ligament

Stabilization of the extensor mechanism may be accomplished by reconstruction of the MPFL in some patients.[14] Amis and associates[15] reviewed current knowledge of the MPFL and noted that the structure is not always identifiable. They reported that the MPFL is most effective in full extension, rapidly losing tension by 20° of knee flexion. A substantial pull on the patella is necessary to reduce it into the trochlea from a lateral tracking position, thereby increasing the risk of adding load to the patella if placing a medial tether (MPFL reconstruction) is used as the sole means of bringing a malaligned patella into normal alignment (Fig. 4). MPFL reconstruction, therefore, should be performed to restore medial balance to the extensor mechanism, particularly in extension, when proper tracking/alignment has been achieved by other means, such as distal realignment. Mini-open MPFL advancement is usually sufficient. Avoiding accentuation of load on damaged or deficient articular surfaces is critical in patients with patellofemoral pain, particularly in those with medial articular lesions. MPFL reconstruction is most effective when there is trochlear dysplasia requiring stabilization of the extensor mechanism beyond what distal realignment can accomplish.

David Dejour has recently modified the technique of trochleaplasty (D. Dejour, MD, Lyon, France, unpublished data, 2004), and this procedure may also be appropriate in a small number of patients with severe trochlea dysplasia.

Distal Realignment

Distal realignment is the most definitive alternative for repositioning the malaligned extensor mechanism. A simple Elmslie-Trillat procedure, accomplished through a short anterior incision adjacent to the tibial tubercle, reestablishes proper patellar tracking and allows early motion[12] (Fig. 5). Cautious proximal reconstruction by mini-open advancement of the medial capsule and vastus medialis or MPFL reconstruction may be considered to add stability in selected cases, particularly when there is trochlear dysplasia and concern about further instability despite distal realignment alone (Fig. 6).

Anteriorization or Anteromedialization of the Tibial Tubercle

Anteriorization or anteromedialization of the tibial tubercle unloads distal and/or lateral patella articular le-

FIGURE 4

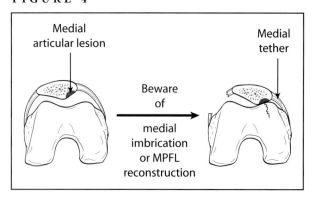

Avoid medial imbrication onto an articular lesion.

FIGURE 6

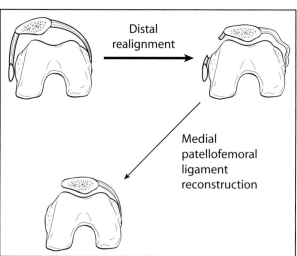

Restore proper tracking first, then provide retinacular support selectively to maintain patellofemoral balance through flexion and extension.

FIGURE 5

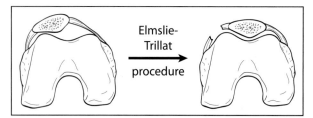

Tibial tubercle transfer can restore a proper relationship between the patella and trochlea by balancing contact stresses.

FIGURE 7

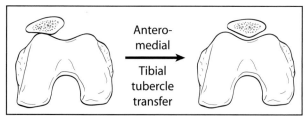

Anteromedial tibial tubercle transfer unloads the lateral and distal patella.

sions at the time of realignment.[12,16-19] With these commonly occuring lesions, the anteromedial tibial tubercle transfer procedure is particularly helpful in gaining long-term relief of patellofemoral pain and instability[12] (Fig. 7). This procedure effectively unloads the frequently painful distal central lesion on the patella.[17] Before moving the patella anteromedially, however, the surgeon should make sure that there is adequate proximal medial patellar articular cartilage (Fig. 8).

Resurfacing of the Medial Patella

Resurfacing of the medial patella with osteochondral autograft or allograft following lateral dislocations that have caused severe damage to the patella may be advised at the time of extensor mechanism stabilization or realignment for recurrent patellar instability.[20] Trochlear lesions may be successfully treated with articular cartilage cell or osteochondral transplantation, sometimes in conjunction with an anteromedial tibial tubercle transfer.

Assessment of Tissue Quality

In patellofemoral realignment surgery, tissue quality should be carefully assessed to determine whether reconstruction of the MPFL or imbrication of the medial capsule is more appropriate.[21] Imbrication should not be used if the tissue quality is poor. Kelly and Insall (M. Kelly, S. Insall, personal communication, 2004) reported that vastus medialis obliquus advancement alone, without medial imbrication, reestablishes patellofemoral balance and minimizes the risk of overloading the medial patel-

FIGURE 8

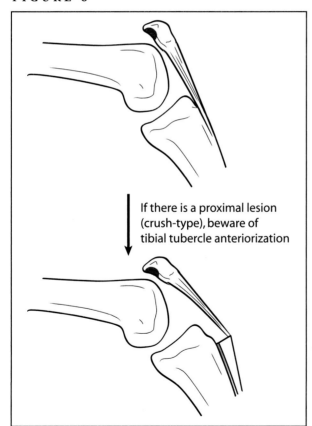

Avoid tibial tubercle anteriorization onto a proximal articular lesion.

FIGURE 9

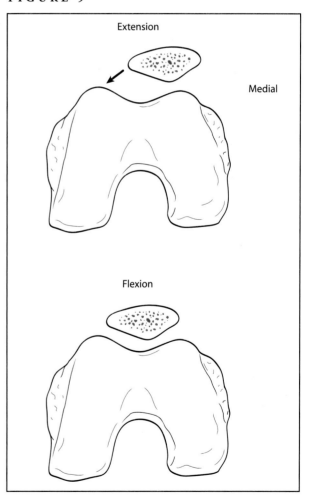

In the patient with medial patella subluxation, the patella jumps suddenly from too far medial back into the trochlea, often with giving way of the knee.

la. Amis and associates[15] reported that repairing the connection of the vastus medialis to the MPFL and adductor tubercle reestablishes proper vastus medialis obliquus functional support of the patella. When choosing a realignment procedure, confirm the existence of a true malalignment,[22,23] and design the surgery to adequately correct the problem but avoid unnecessary repairs. I like to see and palpate the MPFL (or its remnant) to ensure that there is tissue (attached at the appropriate anatomic sites) in this region that will imbricate.

COMPLICATIONS

Medial patellar subluxation (lateral movement of the patella from too far medial back into the trochlea) should be considered as a cause of failure in patients whose condition worsens after undergoing realignment surgery[24] (Fig. 9). This extremely disabling condition, usually worse than the original lateral subluxation, causes very sudden giving way of the knee as the patella jumps back into the trochlea from an overmedialized position. Once identified, medial patellar subluxation usually can be corrected by reconstructing the deficient lateral retinaculum.

CONCLUSIONS

By considering the many factors involved in patellar instability, the surgeon can formulate a logical treatment plan for each patient. Proximal insufficiency should be treated by restoration of proximal retinacular balance. When the alignment vector is off, the surgeon should move the tibial tubercle as needed to balance the extensor mechanism, and then reconstruct proximal retinacular balance as needed. Anteromedial tibial tubercle transfer is appropriate to unload the distal and lateral patella when there are symptomatic articular lesions in these areas.

REFERENCES

1. Dye SF, Staubli HU, Biedert RM, et al: The mosaic of pathophysiology causing patellofemoral pain: Therapeutic implications. *Oper Tech Sports Med* 1999;7:46-54.
2. Fulkerson JP, Arendt EA: Anterior knee pain in females. *Clin Orthop* 2000;372:69-73.
3. Powers CM, Landel R, Perry J: Timing and intensity of vastus muscle activity during functional activities in subjects with and without patellofemoral pain. *Phys Ther* 1996;76:946-955.
4. Wilk KE, Davies GJ, Mangine RE, et al: Patellofemoral disorders: A classification system and clinical guidelines for nonoperative rehabilitation. *J Orthop Sports Phys Ther* 1998;28:307-322.
5. Werner S: An evaluation of knee extensor and knee flexor torques and EMGs in patients with patellofemoral pain syndrome in comparison with matched controls. *Knee Surg Sports Traumatol Arthrosc* 1995;3:89-94.
6. McConnell J: The management of chondromalacia patella: A long-term solution. *Aust J Physiother* 1986;32:215-223.
7. Witvrouw E, Lysens R, Bellemans J, et al: Open versus closed kinetic chain exercises for patellofemoral pain: A prospective randomized study. *Am J Sports Med* 2000;28:687-694.
8. Fulkerson JP, Tennant R, Jaivin JS, et al: Histologic evidence of retinacular nerve injury associated with patellofemoral malalignment. *Clin Orthop* 1985;197: 196-205.
9. Biedert RM, Stauffer E, Friederich NF: Occurrence of free nerve endings in the soft tissue of the knee joint: A histologic investigation. *Am J Sports Med* 1992;20:430-433.
10. Sanchis-Alfonso V, Rosello-Sastre E, Monteaudo-Castro C, et al: Quantitative analysis of nerve changes in the lateral retinaculum in patients with isolated symptomatic patellofemoral malalignment: A preliminary study. *Am J Sports Med* 1998;26:703-709.
11. Witonski D, Wagrowska-Danielewicz M: Distribution of substance-P nerve fibers in the knee joint in patients with anterior knee pain syndrome: A preliminary report. *Knee Surg Sports Traumatol Arthrosc* 1999;7:177-183.
12. Post WR, Fulkerson JP: Distal realignment of the patellofemoral joint: Indications, effects, results, and recommendations. *Orthop Clin North Am* 1992;23:631-643.
13. Fulkerson JP, Schutzer SF, Ramsby GR, et al: Computerized tomography of the patellofemoral joint before and after lateral release or realignment. *Arthroscopy* 1987;3:19-24.
14. Fithian DC, Meier SW: The case for advancement and repair of the medial patellofemoral ligament in patients with recurrent patellar instability. *Oper Tech Sports Med* 1999;7:81-89.
15. Amis AA, Firer P, Mountney J, Senavongse W, Thomas NP: Anatomy and biomechanics of the medial patellofemoral ligament. *The Knee* 2003;10:215-220.
16. Schepsis AA, DeSimone AA, Leach RE: Anterior tibial tubercle transposition for patellofemoral arthrosis: A long-term study. *Am J Knee Surg* 1994;7:13-20.
17. Fulkerson JP, Becker GJ, Meaney JA, et al: Anteromedial tibial tubercle transfer without bone graft. *Am J Sports Med* 1990;18:490-497.
18. Fulkerson JP: Anteromedialization of the tibial tuberosity for patellofemoral malalignment. *Clin Orthop* 1983;177: 176-181.
19. Farr J: Anteromedialization of the tibial tubercle for treatment of patellofemoral malpositioning and concomitant

isolated patellofemoral arthrosis. *Tech Orthop* 1997;12:
151-164.

20. Minas T: A practical algorithm for cartilage repair. *Oper Tech Sports Med* 2000;8:141-143.

21. Burks R, Luker M: Medial patellofemoral ligament reconstruction. *Tech Orthop* 1997;12:185-191.

22. Grelsamer RP: Patellar malalignment. *J Bone Joint Surg Am* 2000;82:1639-1650.

23. Fulkerson J: Diagnosis and treatment of patients with patellofemoral pain. *Am J Sports Med* 2002;30:447-457.

24. Fulkerson JP: A clinical test for medial patella tracking. *Tech Orthop* 1997;12:144.

CHAPTER 3

ROTATIONAL MALALIGNMENT OF THE PATELLA

RONALD P. GRELSAMER, MD

DREW A. STEIN, MD

A correct diagnosis is the key to successful patellar realignment. Before embarking on a surgical or nonsurgical treatment plan designed to address patellar malalignment, two questions must be answered: Is the patella malaligned? and is the malalignment the main source of the patient's pain?

DEFINITION

Patellar malalignment is an abnormal rotational or translational deviation of the patella along any axis.[1] The normal patella lies in the coronol plane, and a line drawn across its medial and lateral borders lies parallel to the popliteal space. Tilting of the patella is a rotational malalignment around the mechanical axis of the leg (or the longitudinal axis of the distal femur).[2] When tilt is present in an unoperated knee, it is always the lateral aspect of the patella that dips posteriorly.

DIFFERENTIAL DIAGNOSIS

Establishing the source of a patient's pain is the greatest challenge. A finding of rotational patellar malalignment does not guarantee that the malalignment is the cause of the pain, as not all patients with patellar malalignment are symptomatic[3] (Fig. 1).

First it must be decided if the pain originates from the knee or is referred from a proximal source such as the hip or spine. Within the knee, a plica, an irritated fat pad, a torn meniscus, or an inflamed synovium can cause anterior knee pain. Pain originating from the extensor mechanism itself may not be related to malalignment; overuse, quadriceps and patellar tendinitis, and tightness of the various musculotendinous groups about the knee are common.[4] More rarely, a patient may have osteochondritis dissecans, a stress fracture, a tumor, or an infection.[5-8]

CHONDROMALACIA

The term chondromalacia, an abbreviation of "chondral malacia," meaning soft cartilage, is mostly of historic interest. The concept of soft cartilage as a pathologic entity dates back to the early 20th century, when it was speculated that cadaveric lesions of the patella accounted for unexplained knee pain among the living.[9] Thus, the term chondromalacia was born. It has been recognized for many years, however, that normal patellar articular cartilage is the thickest and softest in the human body.[10] "Soft" patellar cartilage is therefore normal. Moreover, it

FIGURE 1

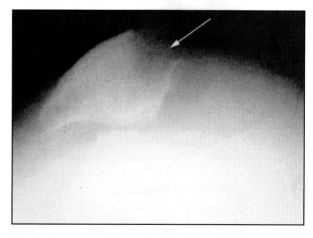

Despite the presence of impressive tilt and lateral displacement indicated by the arrow, the correct diagnosis of this patient's knee pain is diffuse pigmented villonodular synovitis, not malalignment.

has been established that no correlation exists between a chondral lesion of the patella and pain unless the lesion reaches bone and is extensive.[11] Even extensive arthritic lesions in the knee may be asymptomatic, although this premise is controversial.[12] Thus, the term chondromalacia should not be used in the context of patellar pain.

PATHOPHYSIOLOGY

Rotational malalignment of the patella is caused by multiple factors and is not always a source of pain or instability. Anatomic and dynamic factors associated with malalignment have been described from the pelvis on down to the foot, and their clinical expression varies significantly from patient to patient.[13]

Dynamic factors include poor muscle control about the pelvic girdle and thigh; tight soft tissues such as the iliotibial band, hamstrings, quadriceps, and Achilles tendon; and foot pronation.[14] Static factors include lateralization of the tibial tuberosity (which increases the Q angle), a tight lateral retinaculum, a deficient vastus medialis obliquus, trochlear dysplasia, and femoral and/or tibial torsion.[15] It is postulated that these factors increase the lateral patellofemoral forces and/or cause lateral displacement of the patella. In the former case, pain can ensue, whereas in the latter, the patella can become unstable.

Ficat and associates[16] used the term excessive lateral pressure syndrome to describe the painfully excessive pressure borne by the lateral patella in patients with lateral tilting of the patella and a tight lateral retinaculum. In the early 1970s, Ficat and associates[16] in France and Merchant and Mercer[17] in the United States were among the first to advance the concept that malalignment can lead to pain and instability. Tilting may or may not be associated with lateral displacement of the patella[18] (Fig. 2).

Gomori trichrome staining of specimens removed from tight lateral retinacula has revealed evidence of small nerve injury akin to a Morton's neuroma, postulated to result from chronic tension.[19-21] It has been speculated that an excess of substance-P found in some patients with anterior knee pain may cause, potentiate, or trigger patellar pain.[22] Venous congestion has been noted within the patella, and it is conceivable that a tight lateral retinaculum predisposes to such congestion.[20]

The classic pain associated with prolonged sitting may be the result of a combination of stretching of the neuromatous tissue and aggravation of the venous congestion. It may therefore be speculated that the relief of pain following the release of a tight retinaculum may be the result

of the division of injured nerves and the relief of venous congestion.

PATIENT HISTORY

Disorders of the extensor mechanism classically result in anterior pain. As far back as the mid 20th century, however, Karlson[23] in Sweden (1940) and Hughston and associates[24] in the United States (1984) described the association of medial joint pain and tenderness with patellar instability (symptomatic medial-lateral displacement of the patella). Insall and associates[25] also described popliteal pain associated with derangement of the patella.

Pain from rotational malalignment of the patella is typically exacerbated by activity and relieved by rest. It is precipitated by stair climbing, getting up from a seated position, or maintaining the knee in a flexed position for a prolonged period of time ("movie theater sign").

When the patella is unstable, the patient feels the patella slip but is occasionally more aware of the patella's return to a reduced position. Thus, the patient may describe medial displacement when the condition is actually a lateral subluxation. In patients who have undergone patellar realignment surgery, this discrepancy poses a problem for the examiner attempting to determine whether the instability has been under- or overcorrected.

PHYSICAL EXAMINATION

Malalignment can be observed on certain supine, resting patients, whereas in other subjects a dynamic evaluation (eg, jumping, single-leg stance) is required to detect an abnormal alignment.[26] The patient is first asked to stand

FIGURE 2

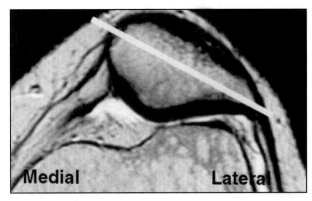

On this MRI scan of an unoperated knee, the patella is tilted with the lateral side down.

and walk. Abnormal foot mechanics are manifested only during ambulation, and abnormal gait patterns may suggest an underlying neurologic condition (eg, Charcot-Marie-Tooth disease, multiple sclerosis). The term miserable malalignment is used to describe the combination of hip anteversion, squinting (inward pointing) of the patella, and external tibial torsion.

When the patient is seated with the leg hanging free, the patella should point directly forward. Any tilt upward indicates that the patella is riding high in the trochlear groove, a clinical sign of patella alta. Examination then includes extension of the knee with the patient seated. Sudden lateral displacement of the patella as the knee nears full extension is called the J sign, or J-tracking, and it signifies considerable subluxation with rotational malalignment, as well as possible trochlear dysplasia or patella alta (Fig. 3).

Joint laxity is assessed at the thumb joint by bringing the patient's thumb toward the forearm and testing for hyperextension at the elbows and knees. Muscle flexibility is initially determined with the patient supine. A pas-

FIGURE 3

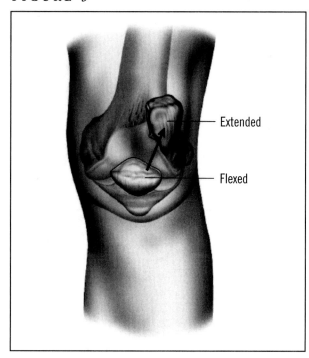

Extended

Flexed

The J sign is a lateral shift of the patella as the knee approaches full extension. *(Reproduced with permission from Grelsamer RP: Patellar pain, in Callaghan J, Rosenberg A, Rubash H, Simonian P, Wickiewicz T (eds):* The Adult Knee. *Philadelphia, PA, Lippincott-Williams & Wilkins, 2003.)*

sive straight leg raise assesses tightness of the hamstrings. Alternatively, the hip is flexed to 90°, the knee is maximally extended, and residual knee flexion is measured with a goniometer.[24] With the knee extended, the ankle is passively dorsiflexed to gauge the flexibility of the gastrocnemius-soleus complex. The Thomas test is used to check for hip flexor contractures. With the patient in the prone position, quadriceps tightness is assessed by asking the patient to pull his or her heel to the buttock. The Ober test, performed with the patient in the decubitus position, assesses the iliotibial band, a common source of anterior knee pain.

Palpation of the soft tissues about the knee is critical and often reveals more important information than any imaging tool.[15] Anterior knee pain is often the result of blunt trauma, such as falling to the ground or striking the dashboard of a car. Such trauma results in a neuroma-like pain from traumatic irritation of the subcutaneous sensory nerves, such as the infrapatellar branch of the saphenous nerve. In these cases, the thumbnail test, where the skin is gently stroked with the thumbnail, elicits focal pain. Similarly, tendinitis or tendinosis of the quadriceps or patellar tendon elicits focal tenderness.

The normal vastus medialis obliquus inserts into the upper third or half of the medial patella and is readily palpable. In patients with patellar malalignment, the vastus medialis obliquus may be dysplastic and virtually invisible, inserting proximal to the superior pole of the patella[27] (Fig. 4).

The medial and lateral borders of the patella are readily palpated using the thumb and index finger, and an imaginary line drawn between these digits should be parallel to the popliteal space (Fig. 5). Tilt (lateral side down) reflects a tight retinaculum, especially if the tilt cannot be passively corrected by the examiner.[28]

Resistance to the examiner's attempt to displace the patella medially is indicative of lateral retinacular tightness. Conversely, excessive lateral displacement reflects incompetence of the medial patellofemoral ligament. These maneuvers are sometimes referred to as the glide test. Attempts have been made to quantify lateral displacement. Some authors divide the patella longitudinally into four quadrants and quantify displacement in units of quadrants, whereas others quantify the glide through instrumentation.[28,29]

When the patella is laterally displaced by the examiner and the patient reports sudden and considerable discomfort as the knee approaches extension, this is termed the

FIGURE 4

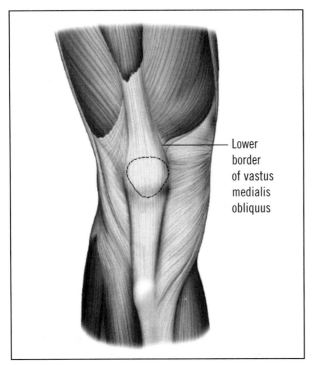

The dysplastic vastus medialis obliquus may barely reach the superior pole of the patella. *(Reproduced with permission from Grelsamer RP: Patellar pain, in Callaghan J, Rosenberg A, Rubash H, Simonian P, Wickiewicz T (eds): The Adult Knee. Philadelphia, PA, Lippincott-Williams & Wilkins, 2003.)*

FIGURE 5

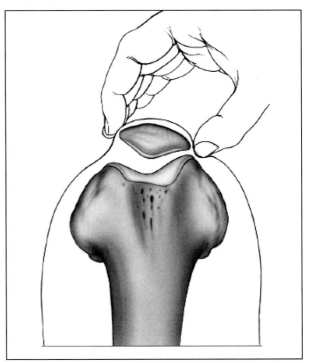

The medial and lateral borders of the patella are readily palpated by the examiner's thumb and index finger. An imaginary line drawn between these digits should be parallel to the popliteal space. *(Reproduced with permission from Grelsamer RP: Patellar pain, in Callaghan J, Rosenberg A, Rubash H, Simonian P, Wickiewicz T (eds): The Adult Knee. Philadelphia, PA, Lippincott-Williams & Wilkins, 2003.)*

apprehension sign. It is present only in patients who exhibit the highest degrees of instability and is therefore not a sensitive test of patellar malalignment.

Palpation of the facets should not elicit pain[25,30] (Fig. 6). The combination of tilt and lateral facet tenderness in the absence of any other positive finding on the physical examination suggests clinically significant patellar malalignment. Whether the facets themselves or the surrounding soft tissues are the true source of pain during palpation remains a subject of debate.

Equally controversial is the role of the Q angle, an indirect measure of the patella's tendency to displace laterally when the quadriceps are contracted.[1,15] The Q angle is usually measured with the knee slightly flexed, and values greater than 20° are considered abnormal. As with all other forms of malalignment, the mere presence of an abnormal Q angle is not an indication for surgery.

Measurement of the Q angle can be awkward because the measurement spans the long area between the anteri-

or superior iliac spine and the tibial tubercle. The tuberosulcus angle is an alternative method of judging the position of the tibial tubercle. With the knee flexed 90°, the tibial tubercle should lie in the midline of the leg. Lateral positioning of the tubercle with this degree of knee flexion is abnormal. Because the extent of the screw-home mechanism varies significantly from patient to patient, however, a tuberosulcus angle may be normal in the presence of an abnormal Q angle.

IMAGING

Imaging should be performed in conjunction with the physical examination, and should not supplant it. Neuromas and tendinitis are not predictably revealed by any common imaging technique, and information pertaining to tilt and displacement of the patella cannot be expected in MRI and radiographic reports.

FIGURE 6

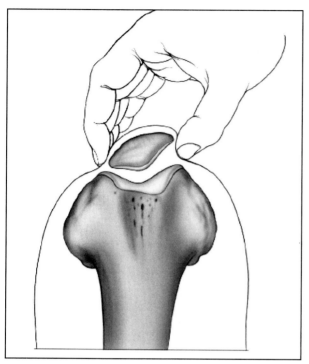

When palpating the facets, tenderness of one or both facets is an abnormal finding. The combination of tilt and lateral facet tenderness in the absence of any other positive finding on the physical examination should suggest to the examiner the presence of clinically significant patellar malalignment. *(Reproduced with permission from Grelsamer RP: Patellar pain, in Callaghan J, Rosenberg A, Rubash H, Simonian P, Wickiewicz T (eds): The Adult Knee. Philadelphia, PA, Lippincott-Williams & Wilkins, 2003.)*

Lateral Radiographs

Radiographs should include a lateral view with the posterior condyles approximated as closely as possible. Quality radiographs allow the clinician to judge the depth of the trochlea through its entire arc.[31] The distance between the lateral femoral condyle and the trochlea is a measure of trochlear depth (Fig. 7, A). The trochlear groove is a major static contributor to patellar stability, and, conversely, the absence of a groove at any point along the trochlear arc is pathologic. The convergence of the bony trochlea and the lateral femoral condyle on a lateral radiograph is termed the crossing sign.[32-34] Milder forms of trochlear dysplasia are proximal and more extensive forms extend distally; therefore, the more distal the crossing sign, the more extensive the dysplasia of the trochlea.

A high-quality lateral radiograph may also reveal abnormal rotational malalignment (tilt) of the patella. The untilted patella features two parallel white lines, one representing the (bony) midline apex of the patella and the other its lateral border. As the patella tilts, the line representing the lateral border of the patella approaches that of the median ridge until the two merge (Figs. 7, B and C).

Axial Radiographs

The axial view should be obtained in the manner described by Merchant and associates[35] but with the knee flexed 30° rather than 45° to better detect abnormal tilt and lateral displacement. Lateral displacement, in particular, is most pronounced in the early degrees of flexion, before the patella engages the trochlear groove. When the radiograph is obtained with the leg in neutral rotation

FIGURE 7

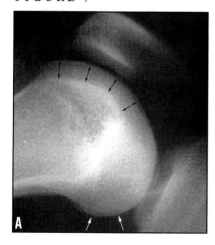

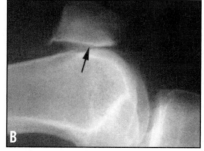

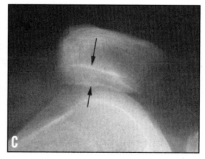

A, On this lateral radiograph of a normal knee, the posterior aspect of the femoral condyles overlap (arrows). The depth of the trochlea can be assessed at every point along its course (two-headed arrows). Tilting (rotational malalignment) of the patella can also be judged. **B,** Lateral radiograph of knee with patellar tilt (black arrow indicates parallel white lines). **C,** Lateral radiograph of knee without abnormal patellar tilt.

FIGURE 8

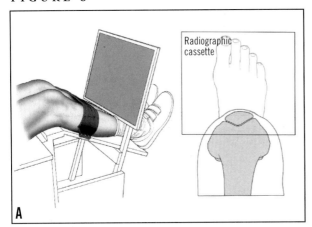
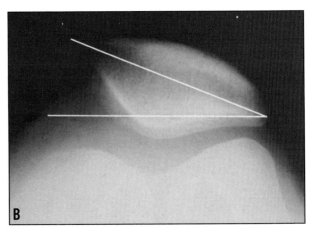

A, Procedure for obtaining an axial radiograph with the leg in neutral rotation, the knee flexed 30°, and the bottom of the radiographic cassette parallel to the ground. **B,** On this axial radiograph, tilt is assessed by measuring the angle subtended by a line connecting the medial and lateral borders of the patella and a horizontal line. A tilt angle greater than 10° is abnormal. *(Reproduced with permission from Grelsamer RP: Patellar pain, in Callaghan J, Rosenberg A, Rubash H, Simonian P, Wickiewicz T (eds):* The Adult Knee. *Philadelphia, PA, Lippincott-Williams & Wilkins, 2003.)*

and the bottom of the radiographic cassette parallel to the ground, tilt is measured by the angle subtended by a line connecting the medial and lateral borders of the patella and any horizontal line (parallel to the bottom of the cassette). Tilt angles greater than 10° are considered abnormal[36] (Fig. 8).

Laurin's lateral patellofemoral angle (LPA) measures the slope of the lateral (bony) facet of the patella relative to a line drawn across the top of the femoral condyles. Any angle that opens laterally is normal.[37] An angle of 0° or an angle that opens medially is abnormal. It is important to recognize that Laurin's study group consisted of patients whose malalignment was so severe they were unstable and required surgery.[37] Thus, the LPA has a high positive predictive value for symptomatic malalignment but is a poor assessment of abnormal tilt. Moreover, the use of a line connecting the top of the condyles is predicated on a normal femoral anatomy, which may not be present in patients with patellar malalignment.

The sulcus angle is formed by the slope of the femoral condyles as they come together to form the trochlea. When the knee is flexed 30° to 45°, the normal sulcus angle is approximately 140°. When the knee is imaged close to extension, the proximal, shallower portion of the trochlea is assessed, and the sulcus angle is smaller. Conversely, with greater degrees of knee flexion, the distal and deeper portion of the trochlea is imaged, and the sulcus angle is larger.[38]

Merchant's congruence angle measures the medial-lateral position of the patella relative to the trochlea and is relatively independent of leg rotation. The congruence angle should be negative, ie, the (bony) apex of the patella should be medial to a line that bisects the sulcus angle.[32,35]

Other indices of patellar tilt or displacement include Laurin's patellofemoral index and lateral patellar displacement,[37] and Cross and Waldrop's patellar index.[39]

Magnetic Resonance Imaging/Computed Tomography

MRI provides added information on the articular cartilage, although some chondral lesions may escape detection. When imaging is obtained with the patient supine and the quadriceps relaxed with the knee in slight flexion, the normal patella should be centered over the underlying femur.[40] When tilt is assessed in the manner of Laurin and associates[37] and Schutzer and associates,[18] using the slope of the lateral facet as the yardstick of tilt, angles of less than than 7° indicate abnormal tilt.

Radionuclide Imaging

A nuclear bone scan provides a measure of bony activity and reflects the presence or absence of homeostasis within the knee.[41] A scan that is focally abnormal about the patella suggests that the patella is a source of pain but does not provide a specific diagnosis.

TREATMENT

Nonsurgical

Most patients with rotational malalignment improve with a nonsurgical program. Failure of an inappropriate nonsurgical program, however, is not an indication for surgery. An appropriate treatment program should include treatment by a dedicated physical therapist and a combination of taping, bracing, medication, and activity modification. Shoe orthoses are advisable in patients with abnormal foot mechanics.

Surgical

Surgery is indicated in the small number of patients with persistent, disabling pain and in patients with recurrent subluxation or dislocation. The need for surgery in patients with a first-time dislocation should be assessed on a case-by-case basis.

The surgeon most commonly focuses on three anatomic areas: the lateral retinaculum, the medial parapatellar tissues, and the tibial tubercle. Surgery on the lateral retinaculum and/or the medial tissues is commonly referred to as a proximal realignment, whereas surgery on the patellar tendon and tibial tubercle is called a distal realignment. Different schools of thought exist with regard to performing one type of realignment versus the other.

Isolated Lateral Retinacular Release

At the time of their seminal description of patellar tilt, Ficat and associates[16] and Merchant and Mercer[17] proposed a surgical cure for this condition: division of the lateral retinaculum. In addition to improving the tracking and pressure distribution within the patella, division of the lateral retinaculum may partially denervate the patella and relieve venous congestion. The popularity of the lateral release has fluctuated as orthopaedists have attempted to determine the true place of this relatively simple operation.[28,42,43] The use of arthroscopic techniques in the 1980s greatly increased the appeal of the lateral retinacular release, to the point where the procedure was performed on patients with anterior knee pain regardless of whether the retinaculum was tight. This led to disappointing results. When these outcomes were combined with the risk of hemarthrosis, which has been reported to occur in up to 10% of patients, some surgeons concluded that the isolated lateral retinacular release is an inferior surgical procedure.[44,45] This opinion is reinforced by reports of early good results followed by late relapses.[43] The literature provides only scant information on the

exact indication for the isolated lateral retinacular release, but an excessively tight lateral retinaculum remains a basic criterion for the procedure.

Technique The original procedure consisted of a long skin incision that encompassed the patella and the tibial tubercle. The lateral retinaculum was divided from the superior pole of the patella down to the most distal aspect of the tibial tubercle, and the synovium was incised. With arthroscopic techniques and the trend toward smaller incisions, surgeons have tended to abandon the division of the retinaculum below the joint line. Through a 1- to 2-cm skin incision anywhere about the lateral patella, the surgeon can effectively divide or lengthen the retinaculum from the superior pole of the patella down to the joint line.[46]

The need for a skin incision can be obviated completely by use of a pure arthroscopic approach[47] (Fig. 9). The

FIGURE 9

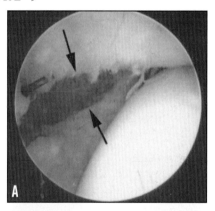
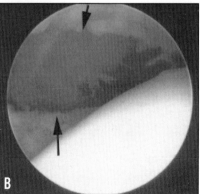

Arthroscopic division of a tight lateral retinaculum. Wide separation of the cut edges is accomplished at the completion of the procedure. **A,** Early phase of procedure. **B,** End of procedure.

retinaculum is approached from inside out or, by way of an instrument passed between the skin and the retinaculum, from outside in. Tourniquet time should be kept to a minimum or not used at all. Hemarthrosis is the principle complication following a lateral release, and the amount of bleeding encountered upon division of the retinaculum will be determined by the precise location of the superior lateral geniculate artery. This artery demonstrates an inconsistent pattern, inserting just above, just below, or just at the level of the superior pole of the patella.[48] Electrocautery used to divide the retinaculum minimizes the risk of bleeding but does not eliminate it. A delayed hemarthrosis may also occur in patients who appear to have had adequate intraoperative hemostasis.

An inadequate release will lead to persistent symptoms, whereas an excessive release may lead to medial instability.[49] Accordingly, the release should not be carried proximally into the quadriceps tendon. A less common but more disastrous complication is division of the patellar or quadriceps tendon. To prevent this complication, a spinal needle is placed into the knee at the top and bottom of the planned release, and the release is performed along a line connecting the two needles.

Plication and Advancement of the Medial Parapatellar Tissues

In certain circumstances, such as particularly severe tilt (>15°), lateral displacement of the patella, or severe vastus medialis obliquus dysplasia, the lateral release should be supplemented with surgery on the medial soft tissues. The surgery itself may consist of plication (open or arthroscopic) or division/advancement of the entire soft-tissue envelope, including the vastus medialis obliquus, the medial retinaculum, the medial patellofemoral ligament, and the synovium. Because these soft tissues pull the patella posteriorly as well as medially, it is important to not overtension these structures.[50] Supraphysiologic tension will lead to abnormal stresses on the medial patella.

Tibial Tubercle Transfers

A medial transfer of the tibial tubercle will diminish the Q angle. Cox[51] reported that medialization of the tibial tubercle (Elmslie-Trillat procedure) may be performed if an abnormal Q angle is part of the pathology. Anterior displacement of the tibial tubercle (Maquet procedure) will diminish patellofemoral stresses, especially over the distal portion of the patella.[52] Accordingly, a combination of medialization and anteriorization as described by Fulkerson[53] will address both an increased Q angle and a distal lesion of the patella, should both be present. A Fulkerson-type osteotomy should be approached with caution in a patient with a trochlear lesion or more diffuse arthritic lesions about the patella.

CONCLUSIONS

Before embarking on a nonsurgical or surgical treatment program, the orthopaedic surgeon must have a more specific diagnosis than anterior knee pain or chondromalacia. A thorough history and physical examination, complemented by appropriate radiographic studies and occasionally CT or MRI, will often provide the clinician with an exact diagnosis to which a specific treatment algorithm can be applied.

REFERENCES

1. Grelsamer R: Patellar malalignment. *J Bone Joint Surg Am* 2000;82:1639-1650.
2. Fulkerson JP: Diagnosis and treatment of patients with patellofemoral pain. *Am J Sports Med* 2002;30:447-456.
3. Grelsamer RP: Patellar pain, in Callaghan J, Rosenberg A, Rubash H, Simonian P, Wickiewicz T (eds): *The Adult Knee*. Philadelphia, PA, Lippincott Williams & Wilkins, 2003, pp 941-950.
4. Dye SF: The knee as a biologic transmission with an envelope of function: A theory. *Clin Orthop* 1996;325:10-18.
5. Obedian RS, Grelsamer RP: Osteochondritis dissecans of the distal femur and patella. *Clin Sports Med* 1997;16:157-174.
6. Peters TA, McLean ID: Osteochondritis dissecans of the patellofemoral joint. *Am J Sports Med* 2000;28:63-67.
7. Orava S, Taimela S, Kvist M, et al: Diagnosis and treatment of stress fracture of the patella in athletes. *Knee Surg Sports Traumatol Arthrosc* 1996;4:206-211.
8. Ferguson PC, Griffin AM, Bell RS: Primary patellar tumors. *Clin Orthop* 1997;336:199-204.
9. Aleman O: Chondromalacia post-traumatica patellae. *Acta Orthop Scand* 1928;63:194.
10. Grelsamer RP, Weinstein CH: Applied biomechanics of the patella. *Clin Orthop* 2001;389:9-14.
11. Dye SF, Vaupel GL, Dye CC: Conscious neurosensory mapping of the internal structures of the human knee without intra-articular anesthesia. *Am J Sports Med* 1998;26:773-777.
12. Thompson NW, Ruiz AL, Breslin E, et al: Total knee arthroplasty without patellar resurfacing in isolated patellofemoral osteoarthritis. *J Arthroplasty* 2001;16:607-612.
13. Fulkerson JP, Arendt EA: Anterior knee pain in females. *Clin Orthop* 2000;372:69-73.

14. Grelsamer RP, McConnell J: *The Patella: A Team Approach.* Gaithersburg, MD, Aspen Publishers, 1998.

15. Post WR: Clinical evaluation of patients with patellofemoral disorders. *Arthroscopy* 1999;15:841-851.

16. Ficat P, Ficat C, Bailleux A: External hypertension syndrome of the patella: Its significance in the recognition of arthrosis. *Rev Chir Orthop* 1975;61:39-59.

17. Merchant AC, Mercer RL: Lateral release of the patella: A preliminary report. *Clin Orthop* 1974;139:40-45.

18. Schutzer SF, Ramsby GR, Fulkerson JP: Computed tomographic classification of patellofemoral pain patients. *Orthop Clin North Am* 1986;17:235-248.

19. Fulkerson, JP, Tennant R, Jaivin JS, et al: Histologic evidence of retinacular nerve injury associated with patellofemoral malalignment. *Clin Orthop* 1985;197:196-205.

20. Arnoldi CC: Patellar pain. *Acta Orthop Scand* 1991;244:1-29.

21. Sanchis-Alfonso V, Rosello-Sastre E, Martinez-Sanjuan V: Pathogenesis of anterior knee pain syndrome and functional patellofemoral instability in the active young. *Am J Knee Surg* 1999;12:29-40.

22. Witonski D, Wagrowska-Danielewicz M: Distribution of substance-P nerve fibers in the knee joint in patients with anterior knee pain syndrome: A preliminary report. *Knee Surg Sports Traumatol Arthrosc* 1999;7:177-183.

23. Karlson S: Chondromalacia patellae. *Acta Orthop Scand* 1940;83:347.

24. Hughston JC, Walsh WM, Puddu G: *Patellar Subluxation and Dislocation.* Philadelphia, PA, WB Saunders, 1984.

25. Insall J, Falvo KA, Wise DW: Chondromalacia patellae: A prospective study. *J Bone Joint Surg Am* 1976;58:1-8.

26. Witvrouw E, Lysens R, Bellemans J, et al: Intrinsic risk factors for the development of anterior knee pain in an athletic population: A two-year prospective study. *Am J Sports Med* 2000;28:480-489.

27. Raimondo RA, Ahmad CS, Blankevoort L, et al: Patellar stabilization: A quantitative evaluation of the vastus medialis obliquus muscle. *Orthopedics* 1998;21:791-795.

28. Kolowich PA, Paulos LE, Rosenberg TD, et al: Lateral release of the patella: Indications and contraindications. *Am J Sports Med* 1990;18:359-365.

29. Hautamaa PV, Fithian DC, Kaufman KR, et al: Medial soft tissue restraints in lateral patellar instability and repair. *Clin Orthop* 1998;349:174-182.

30. Dehaven KE, Dolan WA, Mayer PJ: Chondromalacia patellae in athletes: Clinical presentation and conservative management. *Am J Sports Med* 1979;7:5-11.

31. Malghem J, Maldague B: Depth insufficiency of the proximal trochlear groove on lateral radiographs of the knee: Relation to patellar dislocation. *Radiology* 1989;170:507-510.

32. Aglietti P, Insall JN, Cerulli G: Patellar pain and incongruence: I. Measurements of incongruence. *Clin Orthop* 1983;176:217-224.

33. Dejour H, Walch G, Neyret P, Adeleine P: La dysplasie de la trochlée fémorale. *Rev Chir Orthop* 1990;76:45-54.

34. Grelsamer RP, Tedder JL: The lateral trochlear sign: Femoral trochlear dysplasia as seen on a lateral view roentgenograph. *Clin Orthop* 1992;281:159-162.

35. Merchant AC, Mercer RL, Jacobsen RH, et al: Roentgenographic analysis of patellofemoral congruence. *J Bone Joint Surg Am* 1974;56:1391-1396.

36. Grelsamer RP, Bazos AN, Proctor CS: Radiographic analysis of patellar tilt. *J Bone Joint Surg Br* 1993;75:822-824.

37. Laurin CA, Dussault R, Levesque HP: The tangential x-ray investigation of the patellofemoral joint: X-ray technique, diagnostic criteria and their interpretation. *Clin Orthop* 1979;144:16-26.

38. Brattstrom H, Ahlgren SA: Patella shape and degenerative changes in the femoro-patellar joint. *Acta Orthop Scand* 1959;29:153-154.

39. Cross MJ, Waldrop J: The patella index as a guide to the understanding and diagnosis of patellofemoral instability. *Clin Orthop* 1975;110:174-176.

40. Grelsamer, RP, Newton PM, Staron RB: The medial-lateral position of the patella on routine magnetic resonance imaging: When is normal not normal? *Arthroscopy* 1998;14:23-28.

41. Dye SF, Chew MH: The use of scintigraphy to detect increased osseous metabolic activity about the knee. *Instr Course Lect* 1994;43:453-469.

42. Shea KP, Fulkerson JP: Preoperative computed tomography scanning and arthroscopy in predicting outcome after lateral retinacular release. *Arthroscopy* 1992;8:327-334.

43. Dandy DJ, Desai SS: The results of arthroscopic lateral release of the extensor mechanism for recurrent dislocation of the patella after 8 years. *Arthroscopy* 1994;10:540-545.

44. Flandry F, Hughston JC: Complications of extensor mechanism surgery for patellar malalignment. *Am J Orthop* 1995;24:534-543.

45. Schneider T, Fink B, Abel R, et al: Hemarthrosis as a major complication after arthroscopic subcutaneous lateral retinacular release: A prospective study. *Am J Knee Surg* 1998;11:95-100.

46. Ceder LC, Larson RL: Z-plasty lateral retinacular release for the treatment of patellar compression syndrome. *Clin Orthop* 1979;144:110-113.

47. O'Neill DB: Open lateral retinacular lengthening compared with arthroscopic release: A prospective, randomized outcome study. *J Bone Joint Surg* Am 1997;79:1759-1769.

48. Vialle R, Beddouk A, Cronier P, Fournier D: Prévention des complications hémorragiques de la section du retinaculum patellaire lateral. *Rev Chir Orthop* 1997;83:665-669.

49. Hughston JC, Deese M: Medial subluxation of the patella as a complication of lateral retinacular release. *Am J Sports Med* 1998;16:383-388.

50. Fulkerson JP: *Disorders of the Patellofemoral Joint*, ed 4. Philadelphia, PA, Lippincott-Williams & Wilkins, 2004.

51. Cox JS: An evaluation of the Elmslie-Trillat procedure for management of patellar dislocations and subluxations: A preliminary report. *Am J Sports Med* 1976;4:72-77.

52. Maquet P: Advancement of the tibial tuberosity. *Clin Orthop* 1976;115:225-230.

53. Fulkerson JP: Anteromedialization of the tibial tuberosity for patellofemoral malalignment. *Clin Orthop* 1983;177: 176-181.

MILD PATELLAR INSTABILITY: ARTHROSCOPIC RECONSTRUCTION

JEFFREY L. HALBRECHT, MD

Patellar instability, defined in this chapter as a history of mild to moderate instability that involves at least one actual lateral dislocation of the patella or recurrent lateral subluxation, is a relatively common problem, affecting approximately 43 of 100,000 adolescents per year.[1] Treatment recommendations are controversial and vary widely by geographic region and surgeon. This chapter summarizes and provides updated arthroscopic realignment treatment recommendations for patients with mild to moderate instability. Rarer forms of patellar instability, such as medial, superior, or intra-articular, are beyond the scope of this chapter.

PATHOANATOMY

Patellar stability is determined by a complex combination of factors, including trochlear depth, patellar morphology, Q angle, and the integrity of the medial stabilizing ligaments. The most important retinacular stabilizers are the medial patellofemoral ligament (MPFL), which provides 60% of stability, and the patellomeniscal ligament, which provides 13%.[2]

Several recent studies on acute patellar dislocations have used MRI to localize the damage to the patellar stabilizers that occurs at the time of dislocation.[3] In acute first-time dislocations, most injuries involve disruptions of the MPFL, usually near the femoral attachment. Intrasubstance damage may also occur, however, and in patients with recurrent dislocations and subluxations, chronic stretch of the MPFL is implicated rather than an avulsion (29 of 49 patients had a scarred MPFL still in continuity).[3] These findings are similar to those reported for ankle instability that showed a lax anterior talofibular ligament with intact attachment sites rather than a true avulsion. These studies show that proximal realignment with reconstruction of the medial soft-tissue restraints is an important approach in the treatment of patellar instability.

More than 100 surgical procedures have been described for patellar instability, but many are of historic interest only. Similar to surgical procedures for shoulder instability, the current trend is toward anatomic repairs to restore disrupted structures, rather than reconstruction using imaginative methods and convoluted grafts. Recent studies indicate that repair of the MPFL is an important goal for a successful proximal stabilization; however, how this goal is achieved remains controversial.

THE ARGUMENT FOR SURGICAL TREATMENT

Long-term studies show that the natural history of patellar instability that is managed nonsurgically is poor. Hawkins and associates[4] reported a 20% incidence of ongoing instability and a 15% incidence of pain and crepitus in 20 patients with acute dislocations treated nonsurgically. Cofield and Bryan[5] reported a 44% incidence of redislocation in a series of 48 patients with acute dislocations; 27% of these patients went on to subsequent surgery and, taking into account subjective criteria, 52% were considered failures. McManus and associates[6] reported on 21 patients with acute dislocations treated nonsurgically; 5 had redislocations and 11 remained symptomatic. Cash and Hughston,[7] in an average 8-year follow-up of 100 patients (103 knees), reported a redislocation rate of 20% to 43% depending on anatomic evidence of dysplasia with a predisposition to instability.

Indications for surgical treatment of patellar instability include failure of nonsurgical management, an osteochondral fracture (loose body) following a dislocation, recurring instability, and findings of severe residual malalignment on a postreduction radiograph. Various surgical techniques have been proposed to correct patellar instability.

Lateral Release

Results for lateral release alone have been mixed, with a high incidence of recurring instability.[8-10] Lateral release alone does not address the disrupted anatomy of the medial retinaculum, and most authors do not consider this an effective treatment for true patellar instability or malalignment.[11]

Medial Reefing

When surgery is indicated for patellar instability, most authors recommend some type of proximal soft-tissue realignment. Complex surgical recommendations, such as the extensive open reefing as described by Insall and associates,[12] have fallen out of favor. Minimally invasive open procedures for repair of the medial retinaculum are now the preferred method of repair.[13] Several arthroscopically assisted procedures have also been reported,[14-16] as well as an all-arthroscopic method[17] that is my current preferred technique. Distal bony realignment procedures are reserved for patients with severe malalignment and a high Q angle or for patients in whom previous proximal soft-tissue realignments have failed.

ARTHROSCOPICALLY ASSISTED PROXIMAL REALIGNMENT

Initial recommendations for arthroscopic patellar realignment consisted primarily of arthroscopically assisted techniques using a medial incision. Yamamoto[14] reported on 30 acute patellar dislocations treated with arthroscopic lateral release and arthroscopically assisted repair of the medial retinaculum. He recommended the transcutaneous passage of sutures through the retinaculum using a large curved needle, although the sutures were still tied through a medial skin incision. Only acute dislocations were treated. Results were excellent, with only one case of redislocation.

Small[15] reported on a modified version of the Yamamoto technique, also using an arthroscopically assisted method and a small medial incision. In this study of 24 patients (27 knees), which included those with acute and recurrent dislocations and malalignment and subluxation, results were good to excellent in 92.5% of the knees.

There were two recurrent subluxations, one reoperation for arthrofibrosis, and one superficial infection.

Henry and Pflum[16] described an arthroscopically assisted technique that used cannulated needles but in which the sutures were tied through a medial incision as well. No follow-up series or results were reported.

ALL-ARTHROSCOPIC PROXIMAL REALIGNMENT

Surgical Technique

My current procedure of choice for patients with patellar instability is an all-arthroscopic proximal realignment. Surgery is performed under general anesthesia with a thigh holder in place. A tourniquet is applied but rarely

FIGURE 1

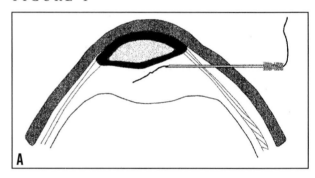

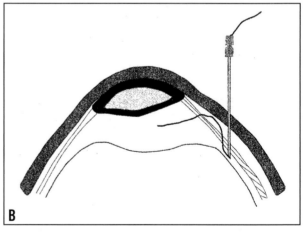

Technique for arthroscopic medial reefing. **A,** A No. 1 PDS suture is passed through a 17-gauge epidural needle that has been inserted percutaneously through the medial retinaculum. **B,** The needle is withdrawn and reinserted through the retinaculum only, without withdrawing through the skin, thus creating an all-inside stitch. *(Reproduced with permission from Halbrecht JL: Arthroscopic patella realignment: An all-inside technique. Arthroscopy 2001;17:940-945.)*

FIGURE 2

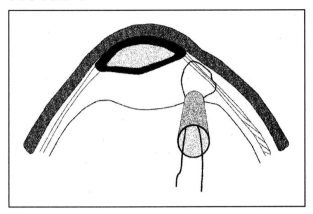

The suture ends are retrieved through the anteromedial portal and tied using standard arthroscopic knot-tying techniques.

FIGURE 3

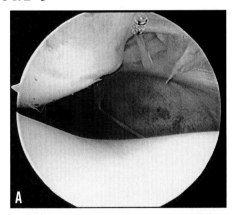

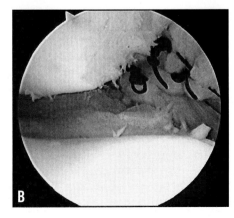

Arthroscopic appearance before (**A**) and after (**B**) all-arthroscopic patellar realignment. Note the appearance of the sutures along the medial retinaculum tied from inside the joint.

inflated. Before plication, a healing response is created along the medial retinaculum by gently shaving with a whisker blade or by using a thermal radiofrequency technique. Medial retinacular sutures are introduced percutaneously using an epidural needle. An epidural needle is essential because the noncutting edge on the inner bevel of the tip prevents cutting of the suture. The needle is placed adjacent to the patella, and a No. 1 polydioxanone suture (PDS) (Ethicon, Edinburgh, Scotland) is passed manually through the needle (Fig. 1, *A*) and retrieved arthroscopically through an accessory superolateral portal. The needle is gently withdrawn from the retinaculum but not out of the skin. The needle is then redirected subcutaneously approximately 2 to 3 cm posteriorly and reinserted through the retinaculum (Fig. 1, *B*). This creates a loop of suture that is retrieved through the same accessory portal. The needle is then withdrawn completely and the process is repeated until four or five sutures are in place. The sutures are retrieved through an accessory proximal lateral portal and clamped for later imbrication of the medial retinaculum. An arthroscopic lateral release is then performed with a standard electrocautery device. Following lateral release, the medial sutures are tied inside the joint from either the proximal lateral or the anteromedial portals (Fig. 2), using standard arthroscopic knot-tying techniques. The arthroscopic appearance of the area before and after the procedure is shown in Figure 3.

Rehabilitation

Postoperative treatment involves a brace locked in full extension for 1 week, followed by physical therapy for 2 to 3 months. After the first week, the brace is unlocked and the patient begins range-of-motion exercises, but bracing is continued for 3 to 4 weeks, until quadriceps strength returns. Patients are not permitted to flex the knee past 90° for 4 weeks but may begin immediate weight bearing in the brace.

Results

In my recent review of results at 5 years follow-up in 26 patients (29 knees), 93% of patients reported significant subjective improvement.[17] The average Lysholm score improved from 41.5 to 79.3 ($P < 0.05$). Pre- and postoperative radiographs were measured for congruence angle, lateral patellofemoral angle, and lateral patellar displacement, and all showed significant improvement postoperatively ($P < 0.05$) (Fig. 4). No complications or redislocations were reported. Patients reported significant im-

FIGURE 4

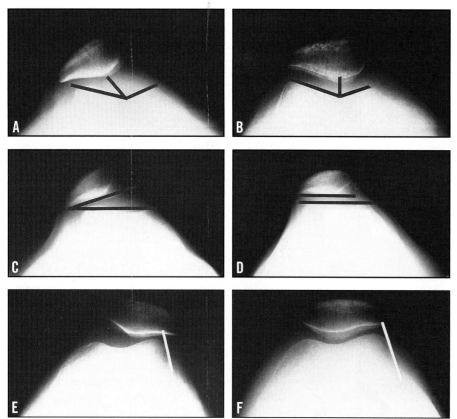

Preoperative and postoperative Merchant view radiographs. The average improvement in the congruence angle was from 30.7° preoperatively **(A)** to 8.2° postoperatively **(B)**. The average improvement in the lateral patellofemoral angle was from –3° preoperatively **(C)** to +9.4° postoperatively **(D)**. The average improvement in lateral patellar translation was from 8.0 mm preoperatively **(E)** to 1.2 mm postoperatively **(F)**.

provements in pain, swelling, stair climbing, crepitus, and ability to return to sports ($P < 0.05$). Although the average Q angle in this study was 11°, I have successfully performed this procedure on patients with Q angles of up to 17°, with no patients requiring reoperation for débridement of scar tissue or manipulation. All patients regained full range of motion compared with the contralateral side.

Although I prefer an all-arthroscopic method of proximal realignment, open and arthroscopically assisted proximal realignment procedures can also effectively prevent recurring instability. However, these procedures may be accompanied by joint stiffness and scar tissue.

DISTAL REALIGNMENT

The goal of the tibial tubercle anteriorization osteotomy described by Maquet[18] was to unload the patellofemoral joint to relieve patellar pain caused by arthrosis. Various authors have modified the original Maquet procedure to include medialization (Elmslie-Trillat) or both medializa-

tion and anteriorization (Fulkerson) to better address malalignment and arthrosis.[19,20] Numerous articles have shown that anteromedialization is effective for painful patellofemoral syndrome associated with malalignment. No clear evidence exists, however, to show that this recommendation is more effective than proximal realignment for patients with moderate degrees of isolated patellofemoral malalignment or instability. In fact, some authors question if the Q angle has any correlation with patellar instability.[21] Some authors who advocate distal realignment actually combine the osteotomy with lateral release[22] or medial reefing,[23] making it difficult to determine if the success of the procedure is the result of the distal or proximal component.

One clear finding is that distal realignment causes complications, and screw removal is requested by about 75% of patients. In a group of 36 patients, many of whom had very complex instabilities and patellofemoral arthritis, 24% required a second surgery,[22] and postoperative fracture was reported in 2.6%.[24] Even nonunions have been reported following distal bony realignment.[25]

This patient population is quite different from those for whom I would recommend arthroscopic patellar realignment.

Although distal realignment can be effective in achieving stability, careful consideration should be given to its use, given its risk of complications and morbidity. In most patients with uncomplicated patellar instability, proximal realignment is sufficient. Distal realignment should be reserved for instability associated with significant articular cartilage degeneration of the patellofemoral joint, in which case anteriorization and medialization has an advantage. Lesser indications for distal realignment include a severe Q angle (> 17°) or failure of arthroscopic proximal realignment.

Conclusions

Arthroscopic proximal realignment is a reliable method of treatment for uncomplicated cases of patellar instability. Early data indicate that properly performed arthroscopic methods offer excellent results with minimal morbidity or associated risks.

References

1. Nietosvaara Y, Aalto K, Kallio PE: Acute patellar dislocation in children: Incidence and associated osteochondral fractures. *J Pediatr Orthop* 1994;14:513-515.

2. Desio SM, Burks RT, Bachus KN: Soft tissue restraints to lateral patellar translation in the human knee. *Am J Sports Med* 1998;26:59-65.

3. Nomura E: Classification of lesions of the medial patellofemoral ligament in patellar dislocation. *Int Orthop* 1999;23:260-263.

4. Hawkins RJ, Bell RH, Anisette G: Acute patella dislocations: The natural history. *Am J Sports Med* 1986;14:117-120.

5. Cofield RH, Bryan RS: Acute dislocation of the patella: Results of conservative treatment. *J Trauma* 1977;17:526-531.

6. McManus MB, Rang M, Heslin J: Acute dislocation of the patella in children. *Clin Orthop* 1979;139:88-91.

7. Cash JD, Hughston JC: Treatment of acute patella dislocation. *Am J Sports Med* 1988;16:244-249.

8. Aglietti P, Pisaneschi A, De Biase P: Recurrent dislocation of patella: Three kinds of surgical treatment. *Ital J Orthop Traumatol* 1992;18:25-36.

9. Dandy DJ, Griffiths D: Lateral release for recurrent dislocation of the patella. *J Bone Joint Surg Br* 1989;71:121-125.

10. Sherman OH, Fox JM, Sperling H, et al: Patellar instability: Treatment by arthroscopic electrosurgical lateral release. *Arthroscopy* 1987;3:152-160.

11. Fulkerson JP, Cautilli RA: Chronic patella instability: Subluxation and dislocation, in Fox JM, Del Pizzo W (eds): *The Patellofemoral Joint*. New York, NY, McGraw-Hill, 1993, pp 135-147.

12. Insall J, Bullough PG, Burstein AH: Proximal tube realignment of the patella for chondromalacia patellae. *Clin Orthop* 1979;144:63-69.

13. Ahmad CS, Stein BE, Matuz D, Henry JH: Immediate surgical repair of the medial patellar stabilizers for acute patellar dislocation: A review of eight cases. *Am J Sports Med* 2000;28:804-810.

14. Yamamoto RK: Arthroscopic repair of the medial retinaculum and capsule in acute patellar dislocations. *Arthroscopy* 1986;2:125-131.

15. Small NC: Arthroscopically assisted proximal extensor mechanism realignment of the knee. *Arthroscopy* 1993;9:63-67.

16. Henry JE, Pflum FA Jr: Arthroscopic proximal patella realignment and stabilization. *Arthroscopy* 1995;11:424-425.

17. Halbrecht JL: Arthroscopic patella realignment: An all-inside technique. *Arthroscopy* 2001;17:940-945.

18. Maquet P: Advancement of the tibial tuberosity. *Clin Orthop* 1976;115:225.

19. Trillat A, Dejour H, Couette A: Diagnostic et traitement des subluxations recidivantes de la rotule. *Rev Chir Orthop* 1964;50:813.

20. Fulkerson JP: Anteromedialization of the tibial tuberosity for patellofemoral malalignment. *Clin Orthop* 1983;177:176.

21. Sanfridsson J, Arnbjornsson A, Friden T, Ryd L, Svahn G, Jonsson K: Femorotibial rotation and the Q angle related to the dislocating patella. *Acta Radiol* 2001;42:218-224.

22. Pidoriano AJ, Weinstein RN, Buuck DA, Fulkerson JP: Correlation of patellar articular lesions with results from anteromedial tibial tubercle transfer. *Am J Sports Med* 1997;25:533-537.

23. Garth WP Jr, DiChristina DG, Holt G: Delayed proximal repair and distal realignment after patellar dislocation. *Clin Orthop* 2000;377:132-144.

24. Stetson WB, Friedman MJ, Fulkerson JP, Cheng M, Buuck D: Fracture of the proximal tibia with immediate weight-bearing after a Fulkerson osteotomy. *Am J Sports Med* 1997;25:570-574.

25. Cosgarea AJ, Freedman JA, McFarland EG: Nonunion of the tibial tubercle shingle following Fulkerson osteotomy. *Am J Knee Surg* 2001;14:51-54.

CHAPTER 5

ACUTE PATELLAR DISLOCATION

WILLIAM R. POST, MD

Patellar dislocation has been well defined as "a clinical entity wherein a traumatic injury disrupts normal or preciously uninjured confinement of the patella within the femoral groove."[1] It is a commonly encountered problem and is sometimes difficult to treat. Some injuries result in rapid recovery without any surgical intervention, whereas others can be catastrophic to a patient's long-term function. The many variables of injury, diagnosis, and treatment have yet to be completely understood. This injury is not rare in orthopaedic practice, but anterior cruciate ligament and meniscal injuries are more common and have been studied more extensively. The purpose of this chapter is to explain the scientific basis and rationale for effective treatment of acute patellar dislocation.

EPIDEMIOLOGY

Fithian and associates[2] reported on 189 patients with patellar instability and found that the risk of primary patellar dislocation was highest for girls between the ages of 10 and 17 years; however, 48% of the patients were boys. Sports injuries caused 61% of the primary dislocations. Few patients had abnormal physical features, contradicting the stereotype of an overweight sedentary adolescent girl.[3]

PATHOANATOMY

Understanding the pathoanatomy of an injury is critical to reach a logical conclusion about treatment. Figure 1 illustrates the medial anatomy of the patellofemoral joint, including the medial patellofemoral ligament (MPFL) and the more distal medial patellotibial ligament. The vastus medialis obliquus (VMO) is reflected superiorly

and normally covers the proximal portion of the MPFL. When the patella dislocates laterally, the MPFL is typically injured. Other injuries which may be associated with lateral dislocation include avulsion fracture from the medial margin of the patella, nondisplaced articular injury, or a potentially displaced articular injury. The MPFL plays an important role in restraint of lateral displacement. In 1993, Conlan and associates[4] reported that the MPFL provided 53% of the restraint in lateral patellar displacement. Burks and associates[5] produced lateral patellar dislocation in a cadaver model and reported that the MPFL

FIGURE 1

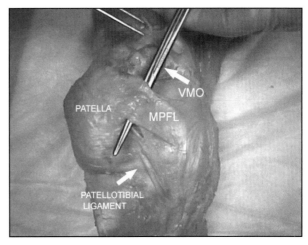

The medial knee dissection illustrates the MPFL attaching to the proximal portion of the patella and the patellotibial ligament attaching more distally. Note the intimate relationship of the VMO to the superior portion of the MPFL. Surgically, the VMO must be reflected from the MPFL for complete exposure, as illustrated here. *(Courtesy of E. Arendt and F. Pena, University of Minnesota Department of Orthopaedics.)*

was injured in 8 of 10 specimens and the patellomeniscal ligament was torn in 6 of 10.

Several clinical studies support these findings. Sallay and associates[6] reported that 15 of 16 patients who underwent surgical exploration after acute patellar dislocation had an avulsion of the MPFL from its femoral origin. Avikainen and associates[7] reported that a femoral avulsion was found in all of their patients who underwent surgical exploration. A separate MRI study of Sallay and associates' patients showed evidence of an avulsion of the MPFL at the adductor tubercle in 19 of 20 patients and increased signal intensity in the medial retinaculum in the area near the patellar attachment in 12 of 20 patients.[8] The latter clearly indicates that approximately 60% of the patients had multifocal injury to the MPFL complex.

In a series of 82 patients with acute dislocations, all of whom had MRI scans within 2 months after injury, Elias and associates[9] reported the following findings: (1) disruptions at the patellar insertion of the medial retinaculum in 76% of patients; (2) injuries at the femoral origin of the MPFL in 49%; (3) injury to the inferior portion of the VMO in 45%; (4) midsubstance injuries in 30% of patients (of these, 92% were partial injuries); and (5) evidence of multifocal injury to the medial stabilizers in 48%.

At present, these studies do not present definitive conclusions about the pathoanatomy of an acute patellar dislocation. This lack of clarity may be the result of different methodologies and radiographic interpretations. What is known from these studies, however, is that the incidence of multifocal injury to the MPFL is significant, even though these injuries do not always occur at the same location or at a single location. Figure 2 illustrates different patterns of medial injury.

Review of MRI scans also reveals a high incidence of osteochondral injury associated with dislocation. Patellar bone bruises or avulsion fractures are present in 28% to 41% of patients, and contusions of the lateral femoral condyle have been documented in 31% to 100% of patients.[6,9-12] Elias and associates[9] reported that 61% of their patients had a contusion of the medial patella, and 80% had an injury to the lateral trochlea. A concave impaction lesion of the distal medial patella, analogous to a Hill-Sachs lesion of the humeral head, was also found in 44%.

PREDISPOSITION TO PATELLAR DISLOCATION

An understanding of the structures that are damaged in an acute patellar dislocation is critical; of equal impor-

FIGURE 2

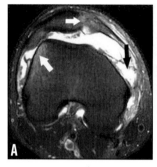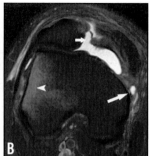

A, MRI scan shows an MPFL avulsion from the medial femoral epicondyle/adductor tubercle area. Note that the most superficial layer of fascia may appear intact, but the ligament is clearly avulsed and displaced anteriorly by hematoma (black arrow). Also note the medial patella and lateral trochlea bone bruises (white arrows). **B,** MRI scan shows that the avulsion originates at the medial border of the patella (short white arrowhead). There is also some injury to the femoral MPFL/VMO origin (long white arrow). A lateral trochlear bone bruise is indicated by the arrowhead.

tance is recognition of a number of factors that may predispose a patient to patellar instability or that ultimately may be of significance for prognostic and/or treatment purposes. One factor that has been well documented to predispose a patient to patellar instability is systemic hypermobility. Dislocation has been reported to occur six times more frequently in patients with systemic hypermobility, whereas articular injury is less than half as likely in these patients.[13,14] In 1969, Beighton and Horan[15] developed easily measurable criteria to identify hypermobility, specifically knee and elbow hyperextension of more than 10° with concomitant fifth finger metacarpophalangeal hyperextension and thumb-forearm apposition. These factors are highly relevant to patient care, and assessing them takes only a few seconds. Articular injury is a major concern associated with possible recurrence of patellar instability; therefore, it is somewhat reassuring to know that patients with hypermobility are much less likely to have a recurrence complicated by osteochondral injury. It is reasonable to conclude that recurrent instability in the setting of hypermobility is less worrisome to long-term function.

Multiple studies have sought to define radiographic criteria that may be important and helpful in understanding patellar instability. A number of factors, including patella alta, a shallow trochlea, lateral patellar tilt, and lateralization of the tibial tubercle, have been shown to increase the incidence of patellar instability. A shallow trochlea and patella alta were both documented by Dejour and associates[16] in 1994. Trochlear depth averaged 2.3 mm in patients with instability compared with an average of 7.8 mm in knees of control subjects. Of patients with patellar instability, 85% had less than 4 mm of trochlear depth. A total of 24% of patients with instability also had a Caton-Deschamps ratio (measurement of patella alta) of more than 1.2 compared with none of the knees in the control subjects.

Laurin and associates[17] reported that the lateral patellofemoral angle was within normal limits in 90% of patients with chondromalacia but was abnormal in patients with lateral patellar instability. Teitge and associates[18] also reported an abnormal lateral patellofemoral angle in patients with lateral patellar instability. Murray and associates[19] demonstrated important radiographic differences in patients with instability, with 98% having a pathologic lateral tilt on the lateral view and 62% having an abnormal lateral translation (subluxation) on the patellar axial view.

Measurement of the tibial tubercle-trochlear groove distance on CT is one way to identify the tibial tubercle in relation to the femoral trochlea. Dejour and associates[16] reported an average of 19.8 mm lateralization compared with 12.7 mm in control subjects. They defined abnormal as greater than 20 mm using this technique.

Linking specific anatomic factors to a predisposition to dislocation (compared with control populations) is of uncertain clinical use because at the present little is known about how these variables affect recurrence after treatment. Establishing a relationship between these anatomic factors and dislocation is simply a means of identifying patients who may be more likely to sustain a first-time dislocation. Additional research is needed to examine differences in response to nonsurgical treatment among patients with predisposing factors. Such studies will need to be very carefully controlled and precise definitions will need to be applied to these factors.

NONSURGICAL TREATMENT

Nonsurgical treatment has been reported to have remarkably consistent results, despite different methods of treatment, duration of immobilization, and length of follow-up. Table 1 presents duration of follow-up, subjective satisfactory results, and recurrence reported by multiple authors.[2,20-24] Maenpaa and Lehto[25] compared redislocation rates in a nonrandomized study of 100 patients treated with cast immobilization, immobilization with a posterior splint, or use of a knee sleeve. After a 13-year follow-up, 37% of patients reported no problems with the affected knee, and 38% to 57% of patients reported redislocation or some other problem. Higher rates of redislocation were associated with relatively less immobilization. In this study, approximately one third of patients reported serious sequelae associated with redislocations. These results suggest that more patients have persistent knee problems even without associated patellar instability. Fithian and associates[2] studied factors in patient history, physical examination, and radiographic and MRI studies and found nothing that predicted recurrence. Patients were entered into the study after a first-time injury or after an injury that was a recurrence. After an acute first-time dislocation, 17% had recurrent stability during the study. Of patients whose instability episode represented a recurrence, 49% recurred during the study. Recurrent dislocations occurred more often in women (70%). Even after 6 months, 58% of the patients with acute dislocation noted limitation in strenuous activity.[3] Therefore, it seems fair to conclude that non-

---

TABLE 1

Nonsurgical Treatment of Patellar Dislocation

Author	Follow-up	No. of Knees	Results	Recurrence
Cofield and Bryan[20]	11.8 years	48	67% satisfied	44%
Hawkins and associates[21]	40 months	20	50% moderate/severe	15%
Cash and Hughston[22]	8.1 years	103	58% good/excellent	29%
Garth and associates[23]	46 months	69	66% good/excellent	26%
Nikku and associates[24]	2 years	55	71% good/excellent	27%
Fithian and associates[2]	2 years	125	Not reported	17%

surgical treatment of patellar dislocation is in need of significant improvement.

SURGICAL TREATMENT

Recurrent dislocation tends to occur less often with surgical treatment than with nonsurgical treatment, although the overall success rates are similar. Good to excellent results range from 58% to 96% with surgical treatment (Table 2) compared with 38% to 57% with nonsurgical treatment (Table 1). Procedures vary, including medial retinacular repair with MPFL reconstruction or augmentation, with or without lateral release. Follow-up in these studies tends to be shorter than studies of nonsurgical treatment.

Several studies are worth exploring in some detail. In a study of 27 patients by Sallay and associates,[6] 19 underwent examination under anesthesia and arthroscopy. Sixteen underwent surgical exploration, and of these, 15 had MPFL tears from the femur and underwent repair. Three underwent a concomitant lateral release because of an exceedingly tight lateral retinaculum, and three had arthroscopic lateral retinacular release without a repair. A total of 12 patients were followed for a minimum of 2 years. Of these, only 58% returned to sports with no or minor limitations, and 42% reported fair results. No patients reported recurrent dislocations, but eight reported intermittent pain and four described having recurrent subluxation.

Ahmad and associates[26] treated eight patients with arthroscopic lateral release, repair of the MPFL at the adductor tubercle, and a VMO repair to the adductor magnus that extended 5 cm above the adductor tubercle. The VMO was displaced anteriorly and superiorly from the adductor magnus origin before repair in all patients. The authors emphasized the importance of MRI in preoperative planning to localize the tear site. Avikainen and associates[7] performed MPFL repair and augmentation without a lateral release in 10 consecutive patients with acute dislocation with a 6-year follow-up. The MPFL was torn from the femur in all of their patients. According to Lysholm criteria, the authors reported zero excellent results, nine good results, and one fair result in a patient who had recurrent instability.

Multiple authors have reported on medial repair, including Vainionpaa and associates[27] who added lateral

---

TABLE 2

Surgical Treatment of Acute Patellar Dislocation

Author	Follow-up	No. of Knees	Results	Recurrence
Dainer and associates[30]	25 months	29/arthroscopy, +/- lateral release	73% good/excellent with lateral release 93% without lateral release	27% with lateral release 0% without
Vainionpaa and associates[27]	2 years	55 medial repair 67% with lateral release	80% good/excellent	9%
Avikainen and associates[7]	6.9 years	10 MPFL augmentation/no lateral release	90% good	10%
Harilainen and Sandelin[29]	6.5 years	53 medial repair/reef 19% with lateral release	60% satisfied	17%
Salley and associates[6]	34 months	MPFL repair, 19% with lateral release	58% good/excellent	≤ 33% subluxated
Nikku and associates[28]	6.9 years	70 medial repair 87% with lateral release 10% lateral release alone	70% good/excellent 96% satisfied	10% 0%
Ahmad and associates[26]	3 years	8 VMO and MPFL repair 100% lateral release		

release in 37 of their 55 patients when they felt the lateral retinaculum was subjectively tight. A total of 80% of their patients had good to excellent results, and the redislocation rate was only 9%. Nikku and associates[28] repaired the medial retinaculum in 70 knees and performed a lateral release in 87% of their patients. The authors reported good to excellent results in 70% of their patients and recurrent dislocations in 10%.

In a study of acute repair, Harilainen and Sandelin[29] reported recurrent instability in 17% of patients and a satisfaction rate of only 60%. As in other studies, a subset of their patients (19%) underwent concurrent lateral release. Dainer and associates[30] treated acute dislocation in 29 patients with arthroscopy alone and included a lateral release in 15 patients. Of interest in this study is that redislocation occurred in 14% of patients, all of whom had had a lateral release. Thus, the importance of lateral release as a confounding variable in previous studies of surgical repair cannot be overemphasized. Such concern is especially pertinent as Desio and associates[31] reported that the lateral retinaculum contributes 10% of the restraint versus lateral patellar translation. Considered together, these results should cause surgeons to seriously reconsider the wisdom of concomitant lateral release in treating patellar instability.

Nikku and associates[28] presented the only study that compares surgical and nonsurgical treatment, and it is considered the best study available that evaluates early surgical repair. A total of 125 patients with acute patellar dislocation underwent arthroscopy, even those reported as receiving nonsurgical treatment. Patients were then randomized to "no repair" and "individually adjusted" proximal realignment procedures followed by rehabilitation. The authors reported no difference in Lysholm criteria or recurrent instability, which occurred in 26% to 36% of the patients. Careful review of all these studies of surgical treatment reveals that there is much room for improvement in both surgical and nonsurgical treatment.

RECOMMENDATIONS

A careful history and physical examination must guide treatment decisions. The physical examination should include assessments for evidence of hypermobility, the presence of a large effusion, specific sites of tenderness between the medial patellar border and the medial epicondyle, and increased lateral patellar translation. Patients with an acute patellar dislocation usually have tenderness along the MPFL. As noted above, the tear most commonly occurs near the femoral attachment of the MPFL. However, more than one site of injury is possible, and injury adjacent to the patella is common. An apprehension sign may not be present; however, this test may stress injured and healing tissue and might be best avoided in the acute setting. Examination for concomitant laxity of the collateral ligaments (especially the medial collateral ligament) or the cruciate ligaments (especially the anterior cruciate ligament) is critical. Complete injuries to the medial collateral ligament with gross patellar instability, though unusual, do occur and merit consideration for early surgical repair.

Evaluation for possible osteochondral injury is critical. Careful attention should be given to radiographs, especially patellar axial views, for evidence of displaced osteochondral fragments. Bone attached to rather large cartilage fragments can be very small so even minor findings on radiographs are of concern. MRI is often a wise choice to evaluate possible osteochondral damage. If surgical treatment is considered, MRI can provide helpful information about the location(s) of ligament and VMO injury.

Minimizing effusion is important to restoring quadriceps control and reducing torn ligament fragments. I believe that immobilization with the patella in a reduced position during the first few weeks of early ligament healing is prudent, as suggested by Maenpaa and Lehto.[25] If the patella is not in a well-reduced position, ligament healing to an appropriate length for future stability could be compromised. In this setting, aspiration of the hemiarthrosis should be considered. If the patella still is not reduced, surgical repair should be considered, even though its efficacy in this situation has not been proved. This problem is unusual in my experience, but one worth anticipating.

Even though we cannot predict which patients will do well with nonsurgical treatment, it seems prudent to use it as an option first. A patient with potentially displaced osteochondral fragments would certainly be the exception. These must be surgically repaired if possible to preserve the function of the articular cartilage.

If immediate surgery is being considered, it is important to remember that an acute medial tear is frequently multifocal. During surgical exploration and repair, the MPFL must be exposed from the medial femoral epicondyle if a single site of injury is not definitely identified on preoperative MRI. In addition, it seems prudent to avoid lateral release and instead focus on restoring normal medial restraint by repairing the MPFL, associated retinacular tissues, and the VMO, which may be torn from its adductor magnus origin. Suture anchors can be useful in repairing femoral and patellar MPFL avulsions. Care should be taken to avoid excessive imbrication of the medial structures, especially in patients with hypermobility or prominent medial patellar osteochondral injury.

Because patients and their injuries differ, it is important to realize that using the same algorithm may not be appropriate for all patients. Certainly, as noted above, patients with hypermobility are less likely to have concurrent osteochondral injury; thus, nonsurgical treatment may be more effective. Lateral release probably should be avoided in acute treatment, based on the study results cited earlier in this chapter, and in all patients with hypermobility. In patients with normal alignment and no predisposing factors who sustain a traumatic dislocation, it is logical to emphasize restoring static restraint in the early stages of nonsurgical treatment by relative immobilization and protection, followed by gradual rehabilitation. Patients with predisposing factors but no hypermobility may be at increased risk for recurrence, although this has not yet been documented in the literature. Underlying mechanical factors such as a shallow trochlea, a lateral tubercle, or patella alta might make recovery from the initial dislocation more difficult. Therefore, increased vigilance in protecting such patients during the early healing phases of an acute dislocation is prudent.

CONCLUSIONS

Both surgical and nonsurgical treatment leave considerable room for improvement; thus, nonsurgical treatment should be the treatment of choice for most patients with acute patellar dislocation. Presently, delayed realignment for recurrent patellar instability has not been proved to be less successful than acute surgery. Likewise, no published evidence currently shows that a second or third episode of patellar instability is any more likely than the first to produce acute, severe, or even catastrophic osteochondral injury. Therefore, I believe it is wise to allow each patient the opportunity to heal without surgical intervention because surgical intervention is available at a later time, with success rates that are similar to or better than those in the acute setting.

It is important to look forward and consider, as a profession, where we should go from here in treating acute patellar dislocations. We need to better understand exactly which patients will do well with nonsurgical treatment.

Some combination of the preexisting anatomy and the pattern of injury may predict the result of treatment. At present, no such data are available. Further research into which rehabilitation and surgical variables are most important to patient success would be welcome and is needed to provide more predictable success to patients with acute patellar dislocation.

REFERENCES

1. Arendt EA, Fithian DC, Cohen E: Current concepts of lateral patella dislocation. *Clin Sports Med* 2002;21:499-519.
2. Fithian DC, Paxton EW, Stone ML, et al: Epidemiology and natural history of acute patellar dislocation. *Am J Sports Med* 2004;32:1114-1121.
3. Atkin DM, Fithian DC, Marangi KS, et al: Characteristics of patients with primary acute lateral patellar dislocation and their recovery within the first 6 months of injury. *Am J Sports Med* 2000;28:472-479.
4. Conlan T, Garth WP Jr, Lemons JE: Evaluation of the medial soft-tissue restraints of the extensor mechanism of the knee. *J Bone Joint Surg Am* 1993;75:682-693.
5. Burks RT, Desio SM, Bachus KN, Tyson L, Springer K: Biomechanical evaluation of lateral patellar dislocations. *Am J Knee Surg* 1998;11:24-31.
6. Sallay PI, Poggi J, Speer KP, Garrett WE: Acute dislocation of the patella: A correlative pathoanatomic study. *Am J Sports Med* 1996;24:52-60.
7. Avikainen VJ, Nikku RK, Seppanen-Lehmonen TK: Adductor magnus tenodesis for patellar dislocation: Technique and preliminary results. *Clin Orthop* 1993;297:12-16.
8. Spritzer CE, Courneya DL, Burk DL Jr, Garrett WE, Strong JA: Medial retinacular complex injury in acute patellar dislocation: MR findings and surgical implications. *Am J Roentgenol* 1997;168:117-122.
9. Elias DA, White LM, Fithian DC: Acute lateral patellar dislocation at MR imaging: Injury patterns of medial patellar soft-tissue restraints and osteochondral injuries of the inferomedial patella. *Radiology* 2002;225:736-743.
10. Kirsch MD, Fitzgerald SW, Friedman H, Rogers LF: Transient lateral patellar dislocation: Diagnosis with MR imaging. *Am J Roentgenol* 1993;161:109-113.
11. Lance E, Deutsch AL, Mink JH: Prior lateral patellar dislocation: MR imaging findings. *Radiology* 1993;189:905-907.
12. Virolainen H, Visuri T, Kuusela T: Acute dislocation of the patella: MR findings. *Radiology* 1993;189:243-246.
13. Runow A: The dislocating patella: Etiology and prognosis in relation to generalized joint laxity and anatomy of the patellar articulation. *Acta Orthop Scand* 1983;201:1-53.
14. Stanitski CL: Articular hypermobility and chondral injury in patients with acute patellar dislocation. *Am J Sports Med* 1995;23:146-150.

15. Beighton P, Horan F: Orthopaedic aspects of the Ehlers-Danlos syndrome. *J Bone Joint Surg Br* 1969;51:444-453.

16. Dejour H, Walch G, Nove-Josserand L, Guier C: Factors of patellar instability: An anatomic radiographic study. *Knee Surg Sports Traumatol Arthrosc* 1994;2:19-26.

17. Laurin CA, Levesque HP, Dussault R, Labelle H, Peides JP: The abnormal lateral patellofemoral angle: A diagnostic roentgenographic sign of recurrent patellar subluxation. *J Bone Joint Surg Am* 1978;60:55-60.

18. Teitge RA, Faerber WW, Des Madryl P, Matelic TM: Stress radiographs of the patellofemoral joint. *J Bone Joint Surg Am* 1996;78:193-203.

19. Murray TF, Dupont JY, Fulkerson JP: Axial and lateral radiographs in evaluating patellofemoral malalignment. *Am J Sports Med* 1999;27:580-584.

20. Cofield RH, Bryan RS: Acute dislocation of the patella: Results of conservative treatment. *J Trauma* 1977;17:526-531.

21. Hawkins RJ, Bell RH, Anisette G: Acute patellar dislocations: The natural history. *Am J Sports Med* 1986;14:117-120.

22. Cash JD, Hughston JC: Treatment of acute patellar dislocation. *Am J Sports Med* 1988;16:244-249.

23. Garth WP Jr, DiChristina DG, Holt G: Delayed proximal repair and distal realignment after patellar dislocation. *Clin Orthop* 2000;377:132-144.

24. Nikku R, Nietosvaara Y, Kallio PE, Aalto K, Michelsson JE: Operative versus closed treatment of primary dislocation of the patella: Similar 2-year results in 125 randomized patients. *Acta Orthop Scand* 1997;68:419-423.

25. Maenpaa H, Lehto MU: Patellar dislocation: The long-term results of nonoperative management in 100 patients. *Am J Sports Med* 1997;25:213-217.

26. Ahmad CS, Stein BE, Matuz D, Henry JH: Immediate surgical repair of the medial patellar stabilizers for acute patellar dislocation: A review of eight cases. *Am J Sports Med* 2000;28:804-810.

27. Vainionpaa S, Laasonen E, Patiala H, Rusanen M, Rokkannen P: Acute dislocation of the patella: Clinical, radiographic and operative findings in 64 consecutive cases. *Acta Orthop Scand* 1986;57:331-333.

28. Nikku R, Nietosvaara Y, Kallio PE, Aalto K, Michelsson JE: Operative versus closed treatment of primary dislocation of the patella: Similar 2-year results in 125 randomized patients. *Acta Orthop Scand* 1997;68:419-423.

29. Harilainen A, Sandelin J: Prospective long-term results of operative treatment in primary dislocation of the patella. *Knee Surg Sports Traumatol Arthrosc* 1993;1:100-103.

30. Dainer RD, Barrack RL, Buckley SL, Alexander AH: Arthroscopic treatment of acute patellar dislocations. *Arthroscopy* 1988;4:267-271.

31. Desio SM, Burks RT, Bachus KN: Soft tissue restraints to lateral patellar translation in the human knee. *Am J Sports Med* 1998;26:59-65.

CHAPTER 6

RECURRENT PATELLAR DISLOCATION

JACK T. ANDRISH, MD

This chapter describes an approach to the treatment of recurrent patellar instability that considers the unique features and expectations of the patient rather than using a generic algorithm. Although an approach that includes an in-depth analysis of the patient's unique pathoanatomy and variations of lower extremity motion is more satisfying than the alternative and would seem to be intellectually defensible,[1] to date its advantages are unsubstantiated. No data exist, however, that would suggest that the customized approach described in this chapter produces results inferior to those achieved by the generic approach and the intellectual satisfaction is far greater.

To develop a treatment approach that accounts for the unique features of the patient with recurrent patellar dislocations, an understanding of how neuromuscular, ligamentous, and morphologic variations of the lower extremity contribute to patellar stability or instability is required. Treatment can then be designed to address the pathologies of form and function rather than to compensate for those abnormalities by creating secondary pathoanatomies.

EPIDEMIOLOGY AND NATURAL HISTORY

In a prospective study of a Kaiser Health Plan population, individuals in their second decade of life had the highest incidence of acute patellar dislocation, with 69% of all dislocations that occurred in a year affecting these individuals. The overall risk for members of this health plan for all ages was 7 per 100,000 per year, but the risk for those between the ages of 10 to 19 years was 31 per 100,000 per year, with a nearly equal distribution among girls and boys (33 per 100,000 per years versus 30 per 100,000 per year, respectively).[2]

Female sex, a family history of patellar instability, and a history of patellar subluxation or dislocation have all been associated with higher risk of subsequent dislocation.[2,3] Furthermore, the degree of trauma associated with the first dislocation is an important indicator of subsequent dislocation.[2] Fithian and associates[2] note that in patients with MRI-documented disruption of the medial retinaculum and the medial patellofemoral ligament (MPFL), the incidence of subsequent patellar dislocation was actually lower than in patients without retinacular injury. This finding is understandable if one considers that patellar dislocation in the absence of MPFL trauma may be indicative of coexisting patellofemoral dysplasia. Crosby and Insall[4] reported that episodes of patellar subluxation/dislocation decreased with time, and the incidence of patellofemoral osteoarthritis was low and not related to the frequency of dislocations.

BIOMECHANICS OF PATELLAR INSTABILITY

Patellar motion is affected by the complex interaction of muscles, ligaments, bone morphology, and lower extremity alignment.[5,6] The retinacular patellofemoral ligaments are important stabilizers of the patella, and, in particular, the MPFL is the primary soft-tissue restraint to lateral translation of the patella during the initial 20° to 30° of knee flexion.[7-11] This ligament is most taut in full extension, with the quadriceps contracted, and assists in guiding the patella into the trochlea during the early stages of flexion.[12] Amis and associates[12] and Senavongse and associates[13] demonstrated that the least resistance to lateral translation of the patella occurs at 20° of flexion, with increasing resistance occurring with further extension and flexion. Once engaged in the trochlea, the patellofemoral joint compression provided by the increasing force vectors of the quadri-ceps and patellar tendons, combined with patellofemoral joint geometry, provides the major effect on stability as knee flexion progresses.[14-16] While the patella is tracking within the trochlea, the slope of the lateral facet of the trochlea provides the main resistance to lateral patellar translation.[17,18] Studies have been conducted on the influence of the musculature and the vastus medialis obliquus (VMO) in particular on knee stability.[19-21] The evidence supporting the VMO as a major determinant in patellofemoral stability is controversial, but as with the retinacular patellofemoral ligaments, the VMO exerts its greatest influence on patellar alignment during the initial stages of knee flexion.[21,22]

Several studies have examined the influence of lower extremity alignment on patellar instability.[16,23-26] Fithian and associates[11] demonstrated, however, that lower extremity and patellofemoral alignment cannot by themselves produce an episode of patellar dislocation without the coexistence of an insufficiency of the soft-tissue restraints by either hyperelasticity or injury.

PATIENT HISTORY

Chronic recurrent dislocations and subluxations of the patella are often more disabling to the patient than isolated ligamentous instability of the knee, and they are certainly more disabling than instability associated with injury to the anterior cruciate ligament (ACL). The difference is that instability that is the result of a torn ACL is typically symptomatic during sport activity. Although this is a significant concern for the active individual, only 15% to 30% of patients with torn ACLs experience instability symptoms with activities of daily living.[27-30] Conversely, patellar instability is typically associated with the knee giving way unexpectedly with minimal trauma during activities of daily living. This sometimes results in significant secondary injuries from falls, and understandably, these patients are frequently extremely apprehensive.

Another important distinction to be made from the history is the patient's perception of the relative importance of the pain. Patellar dislocations are painful, but the pain is secondary to the event. The patient who reports knee pain as the primary problem, with patellar instability events as secondary ("My knee hurts all of the time,

and sometimes it gives out on me."), is viewed differently from the patient whose instability is the primary reason for the consultation ("My knee hurts, but the main reason I am here is that when my patella slips out, the pain is severe."). Good orthopaedic tools exist to manage instability (and the pain that is secondary to the events resulting from instability), but treatment of chronic knee pain or chronic pain associated with patellar instability becomes more difficult. There are multiple causes of chronic knee pain, and not all are structural in nature.[31]

Finally, age at onset and the magnitude of trauma eliciting the patellar dislocation are important. If a significant trauma such as a contact injury in sport (valgus, external rotation of the tibia versus a direct lateralizing blow to the patella) is the first event that produced a patellar dislocation and if the soft-tissue and joint reaction to this trauma is severe, it is likely that the inherent stability of the patella was normal at the time of injury and that closed or open management will be successful unless a significant osteochondral fracture complicates the outcome. On the other hand, if the event was trivial, such as a minor twist or pivot, then it is likely that the patient has one or a combination of pathoanatomies (dynamic and/or static) that predisposed the knee to the first episode and will subsequently contribute to recurrent episodes. In these patients, closed management is frequently insufficient, and even surgical management may result in failure unless the unique features that allowed for the dislocation are adequately addressed.[32]

PHYSICAL EXAMINATION

Physical examination of the patient with chronic recurrent dislocations of the patella involves an awareness of the whole individual. The patient may be apprehensive. The gait may be somewhat unusual, as these patients often use innovative adaptive mechanisms to avoid further episodes. Typically, the patient shows significant apprehension with attempted palpation of the patella, especially with assessment of medial and lateral patellar translation. The examination may be divided into assessments made with the patient standing, walking, sitting, lying supine, lying prone, and lying on the side.

Standing

James and associates[33] first coined the term miserable malalignment syndrome. This finding consists of a kneeing-in posture, or "squinting" patellae, coexisting with proximal tibia vara, medial femoral torsion, an increased

Q angle, and either hyperpronation of the foot, external tibial torsion, or both.[33] Although this lower extremity posture is often found in patients with anterior knee pain, it may be part of a series of anatomic variances associated with but not necessarily causative of patellar instability.

Walking

Not all abnormalities that contribute to patellar instability are static deformities. The dynamics of the patient's gait may demonstrate pathomechanics unique to the individual that predispose to patellar malalignment and instability. The gait most often associated with patellofemoral dysfunction is the kneeing-in gait. This is frequently described as being secondary to medial femoral torsion (femoral anteversion), but it can just as easily be secondary to external tibial torsion, hyperpronation of the foot, or some combination of all three.[34] Kneeing-in is significant because the internal rotation and valgus thrust generates an external rotation moment about the knee with a resultant lateral force on the patella.[16] Although this gait is most frequently associated with the static deformities described above, it may be dynamically induced by altered neuromotor coordination, as in spasticity, or it may be a result of instability of the core musculature of the back, abdomen, and hip.[35,36]

Sitting

With the patient in the seated postion with the knees at the edge of the examining table, assessment of the relative height of the patellae may reveal patella alta or patella baja.[37] The Q angle obtained while the patient is sitting may be more meaningful than when the patient is lying supine because most often the patella is centered in the trochlea at 30° to 90° of flexion.[38-40] With the knee in full extension, however, the patella may be laterally positioned, thus giving the illusion of a normal Q angle. To measure the Q angle in the sitting position, drop a plumb line from the center of the patella. The line should bisect the tibial tuberosity. If the tuberosity is lateral to this line, an abnormally increased Q angle exists.[39,40]

Active knee extension may elicit patellofemoral crepitus suggestive of articular surface injury or degeneration. An extensor lag may signify significant weakness of the quadriceps mechanism, or it may be the result of severe patellar instability with obligatory subluxation or even dislocation with active extension. The J sign or J-tracking is frequently associated with patella alta or trochlear dysplasia.

Medial subluxations or even dislocations of the patella may be difficult to detect without stress radiography, although using the Fulkerson relocation test can be helpful. In this test, the knee is passively supported in extension and the patella is gently subluxated medially.[41] Then the knee is gently flexed while allowing the patella to relocate. If this maneuver results in sudden pain and/or apprehension and especially if the patient relates the sensation to his or her presenting symptoms, the diagnosis of medial patellar subluxation should be considered. Finally, with the patient in the sitting position, the upper extremities can be examined for signs of generalized laxity.[42,43]

Lying Supine

With the patient in the supine position, the examiner can observe, palpate, and test for knee stability as well as joint motion and irritability (the hip as well as the knee). The relative girth and development of the quadriceps and asymmetric or significant atrophy of the VMO may be observed. Effusion may be detected from observation alone, but palpation further quantifies the extent. Palpation also detects areas of retinacular tenderness, and patellofemoral compression may provoke crepitus and/or pain. Patellar mobility is assessed both with the knee fully extended and then with the knee flexed 30°.[44-47] Significant apprehension with passive subluxation is indicative of clinical subluxations. Hypermobility of the patella may confirm the clinical suspicion of patellar subluxations and dislocations, whereas the absence of hypermobility may be even more meaningful because it suggests other possibilities for symptoms of giving way. The presence of a firm end point when lateral stress is applied to the patella, combined with limited translation (two quadrants or less), mitigates against the diagnosis of patellar instability.[32] The supine examination should also include general assessment and documentation of collateral, capsular, and cruciate stability.

Lying Prone

The prone position is best used for detection of femoral and tibial torsion as well as quadriceps contracture. This position allows maintenance of hip extension while flexing the knee to observe the heel-to-buttock distance. Involuntary pelvic tilt and hip flexion during this maneuver indicates tightness of the rectus femoris (Ely test).[36] Inability to fully flex the knee may indicate quadriceps contracture or (painful) internal derangement of the knee.

The transmalleolar axis of the ankle is most relevant to tibial torsion (normally externally rotated 15°), whereas measurement of the amount of internal and external rotation of the hip reveals abnormalities of femoral torsion. The foot position also suggests variations in tibial torsion, but it is important to account for pes planus because the abducted foot position may be confused with external tibial torsion.

Side Lying

This final position is best used to detect contracture of the iliotibial tract (Ober's test). In the Ober test, the knee and hip are flexed. Holding the knee in flexion, the hip is abducted and then extended (holding the knee flexed). The hip is then allowed to adduct. A tight iliotibial band will prevent adduction of the hip in this position. The side lying position also can be used to detect (iatrogenic) medial patellar subluxation as described by Nonweiler and DeLee.[48]

RADIOGRAPHIC FINDINGS

Many authors have described variations in patellar alignment and patellofemoral morphology that may relate to patellar instability,[38,49-51] specifically, those that could be implicated as risk factors for dislocation. Although the order of importance varies among the studies, patella alta and trochlear dysplasia have been identified consistently as important factors associated with recurrent patellar dislocations.[38,49,52-54] Other factors are patellar tilt and increased lateralization of the tibial tuberosity in relation to the trochlear groove.[55,56] Although Dejour and associates[49] believed that patellar tilt was indicative of quadriceps dysplasia, Arendt and associates[32] and Beasley and Vidal[57] related this to insufficiency of the MPFL, which some have implicated as the essential lesion involved in recurrent patellar instability.

Radiographs remain important in the evaluation of patients with patellar instability. Although CT has been viewed as a more sensitive indicator of patellar malalignment because of the ability to obtain axial images in the more provocative degrees of knee flexion (at and near full extension), Murray and associates[58] demonstrated that true lateral radiographs provide similar information. Specifically, the AP view provides an assessment of femoral-tibial alignment and arthrosis, and the lateral view provides an assessment of patellar height, tilt, subluxation, and arthrosis.[59] The depth of the trochlear sulcus as well as variations of dysplasia of the distal femur are all readily identified. The axial view, as described by Laurin and associates[60] and by Merchant and associates,[61] adds to our understanding of trochlear shape and patellar position.

Patella alta is frequently associated with patellar instability; therefore, assessment by radiography is important. Although the Insall-Salvati index and the measurement described by Caton and associates are popular measurements of the patellar height, the index described by Blackburne and Peel is more reproducible.[59]

CT provides important views of patellofemoral alignment and congruence in the early stages of knee flexion, but MRI can provide the same information and has the added advantage of demonstrating the articular cartilage.[18,51,56,62,63] Staubli and associates[63] demonstrated that the contour of the articular cartilage of the patellofemoral joint does not always follow the contour of the subchondral bone. Therefore, it is possible for CT images to appear to show patellofemoral incongruence when indeed the MRI scan reveals true articular congruence. Furthermore, recent demonstrations of dynamic MRI suggest additional advantages in the evaluation of patellofemoral dysfunction.[64] Nevertheless, the extensive database of CT measurements and the efficiency of time and expense for CT versus MRI justify its continued use in the evaluation of patellofemoral alignment.

HISTORIC TREATMENT OPTIONS AND OUTCOMES

Nonsurgical

Nonsurgical management of patellar dislocations has resulted in redislocation rates of 15% to 44% with persistent symptoms of anterior knee pain, instability, and limitations of activity affecting more than 50% of patients.[65-67] Although nonsurgical management protocols vary widely, those including early mobilization have resulted in poorer outcomes.[67,68]

Surgical

The literature describes more than 100 different surgical approaches for recurrent patellar dislocation;[69-74] however, variations in reporting and study design make comparisons among these studies almost impossible. Traditionally, surgical regimens have been one of three types: proximal realignment, distal realignment, or combined. In studies comparing efficacy of proximal versus distal alignment, distal shows no benefit over proximal.[75] Lateral retinacular release as an isolated procedure for patellar instability has been shown to have inferior outcomes.[75,76]

Finally, studies comparing surgical and nonsurgical treatment of patellar instability have failed to show superior long-term clinical results with surgical treatment.[77,78] Some studies of surgical treatment have even shown an increased risk of developing patellofemoral arthrosis despite the reduction in dislocations after surgery.[79-84]

My Preferred Management

The knee is a coupled mechanical system in which a change to any one part of the system affects the other parts of the system.[85] For example, a tibial tuberosity transfer may affect joint loading within the patellofemoral and tibiofemoral joints. Medial transfer of the tibial tuberosity increases joint loading within the medial tibiofemoral compartment and the medial facet of the patellofemoral joint as well as inducing variable changes within the lateral tibiofemoral compartment.[86] Therefore, medialization of the tibial tuberosity should be used cautiously in the varus knee and, if possible, avoided in the medial menisectomized knee. Anteriorization of the tibial tuberosity decreases patellofemoral contact pressures in general; however, the transfer of those forces to a more proximal location on the patella may result in increased loading in those areas.[87] Therefore, anteriorization and anteromedialization of the tibial tuberosity should be used only after recognizing the patellar wear patterns, and they should be avoided when the resultant loads are increased over areas of severe articular cartilage degeneration.[88]

Nonsurgical

Despite the disability that results from recurrent patellar dislocations, persistence with nonsurgical treatment is warranted when the dislocations are isolated or infrequent, not habitual or obligatory, and, most importantly, when the existing patellar mechanics are able to accommodate the rehabilitation process. When the patella dislocates painfully with each attempt at active knee extension, it is often better to perform the realignment first and then begin pelvifemoral rehabilitation once the patella is well aligned and stable.

A rehabilitation program may be successful in the patient who has a history of a series of isolated patellar dislocations that occasionally affect work or play, but in whom there are no overriding mechanical or intra-articular reasons to proceed immediately with a surgical procedure.[89] Pelvifemoral rehabilitation is based on a philosophy of providing core stability through strengthening of the anatomic core musculature (hip, abdomen, back) in addition to the traditional quadriceps progressive resistance exercises.[90] Although the VMO is an important component of patellar stability, its role as the main dynamic stabilizer has been overstated.[21,22,91-93] Weakness of the anatomic core musculature may allow for excessive medial femoral rotation and knee valgus that may contribute or predispose to patellar dislocation or subluxation.[16] Therefore, we initiate and monitor the rehabilitation process for compliance and outcome, and, most importantly, we emphasize to the patient and his or her family that the exercise program is to be continued over the long term to ensure continuing optimal function.

For patients who desire an orthosis, there are several good choices, although the literature lacks evidence-based support.[94-96] For uncomplicated patellar subluxation, I prefer the simple Neoprene J brace. For the patient with significant instability symptoms who wishes to remain active in sports, and especially if there is a component of hypermobility, the TruePull brace (Donjoy Ortho, Vista, CA) designed by Fulkerson has been well tolerated. For the patient with a significant J sign, the Breg patellar tendon orthosis (PTO Neoprene) (Breg Inc, Vista, CA) offers at least a theoretic advantage by exerting a restraining force against lateral displacement, which is greater in extension than in flexion. If a brace is used in the nonsurgical treatment of patellar instability, however, we emphasize that the brace is an adjunct to, not a substitute for, the rehabilitation process.

Surgical

Rather than describing common surgical procedures used for the treatment of patellar instability, I prefer to abandon the "procedure" mentality in favor of an "identify and address the pathoanatomy" approach. I consider a surgical procedure based on whether it addresses an existing pathoanatomy that allows or provokes episodes of patellar subluxation or dislocation. It is possible to identify the anatomic variances unique to the individual as we have discussed[62,97] (Table 1). And so, my first principle in designing a treatment for patellar instability is to individualize, customize, and normalize. My preference is to correct the offending pathoanatomy, not create a secondary pathoanatomy to compensate for the primary pathoanatomy. In choosing a procedure, however, I consider the risk versus the benefit of the individual procedures. Soft-tissue proximal realignment has been shown to be as effective as distal realignment in the treatment of patellar instability.[75]

This approach requires careful and thorough patient evaluation before surgery that includes assessment of

T A B L E   1

Pathoanatomies of Patellar Instability

Trochlear dysplasia

Patella alta

Increased Q angle

Increased TT:TG distance

    Tibial tuberosity:Trochlear groove

Medial patellofemoral ligament insufficiency

VMO hypoplasia/dysplasia

Vastus lateralis dominance

Contracture

    Lateral retinaculum

    I-T band

    Rectus femoris and/or vastus lateralis

        Congenital patellar dislocations

        Obligatory patellar dislocations

Lower extremity malalignment

    Torsion

        Femur, medial

        Tibia, lateral

    Genu valgum

Gait

    Valgus thrust

    Valgus/internal rotation thrust

    Excessive medial rotation of the femur with increased

        external rotation torque of the knee

            Medial femoral torsion

            External tibial torsion

            Excessive foot pronation

            "Core" instability

lower extremity alignment, patellar position and mobility, quadriceps balance, and gait. It also requires a careful radiographic assessment of patellofemoral joint morphology and alignment. I then plan for the method of anesthesia to be used. I prefer to use selective epidural anesthesia or local anesthesia and monitored anesthesia control because it allows the patient to actively extend the knee on command during the surgery. This method is useful when rebalancing the extensor mechanism, and is invaluable in patients with obligatory patellar dislocations that either occur with active knee extension or, in some patients, with knee flexion. It is desirable and helpful for patients with a prominent J sign and lateral pull.

After identification of the pathoanatomies, I consider the risk versus the benefit of the surgical correction of these components. The correction of bone shape and/or alignment by osteotomy can be compelling, but the use of this procedure should be weighed against potential risks of overcorrection, undercorrection, delayed union or nonunion, late fracture, and pathologic changes in joint loading.[24,85,86,98,99] Nevertheless, for some patients the most appropriate surgical tool is an osteotomy.

Soft-tissue realignment and/or reconstruction may be perceived by some as safer, but it requires a high level of surgical expertise and experience.[2] Even then, the potential exists to make the repair/reconstruction too tight. The goal of realignment of the extensor mechanism is to re-establish the balance of forces that results in patellar stability while also maintaining physiologic motion. Stability should not be achieved through overconstraint. Although I recognize the importance of the medial retinacular ligaments and the MPFL, in particular, in enabling the consistent and safe engagement of the patella into the femoral trochlea during the initial 10° to 30° of knee flexion, I do not depend on the MPFL to hold the patella in place. If I use that philosophy (and I have in the past), the potential exists to make the repair/reconstruction too tight. This may result in pain, stiffness, and potential patellofemoral joint overload. The other risk with patellar realignments that rely too heavily on MPFL repair or reconstruction to hold the patella in place while other pathoanatomies affecting alignment are not corrected is the eventual stretching and subsequent incompetence of the procedure. Based on these factors, I prefer to make the medial repair/reconstruction one of the last components of the procedure. After realigning the patella through some combination of osteotomy of the tibial tuberosity, distal femur, and/or lengthening of the lateral retinaculum and/or quadriceps components (vastus lateralis, rectus femoris), the MPFL is either identified and retensioned or reconstructed as needed.

Although proximal patellar realignment has been described, I will elaborate on a few details. The lateral retinaculum contributes to lateral and medial patellar stability.[8,100] The creation of iatrogenic medial instability of the patella is uncommon but not rare.[37,99,101] To release the lateral retinaculum in the presence of patellar instability risks further destabilization of an already unstable joint.[2,13] If the lateral retinaculum is a pathoanatomy by virtue of contracture, then lengthening is preferred over release. Larsen and associates[102] described a method of lateral retinacular lengthening that helps avoid the potential complication of medial patellar subluxation. In some patients, symptomatic patellar hypermobility has responded to reconstruction of a previously released lateral retinaculum.[103]

Surgically balancing the actions of the vastus lateralis and the VMO can be a challenge because the VMO commonly is dysplastic. It can be severely atrophic and/or more vertically oriented rather than oblique. VMO advancement traditionally has been included in proximal realignment, but advancement over the patella does little to increase its mechanical effectiveness. At times, detachment of the VMO to advance it distally over the patella can actually impair its effectiveness by reducing the obliquity of its fibers. It is more advisable to advance the posteromedial corner of the VMO tendon as described by Ahmad and associates[104] to increase its obliquity and mechanical advantage. That said, the vastus lateralis is generally a larger muscle than the VMO with a total cross-sectional area of the quadriceps of 40% compared with 25% for the VMO.[91] Also, a less often described portion of the vastus lateralis is comparable to a vastus lateralis obliquus. When the lateral retinaculum is lengthened rather than released, this oblique portion of the lateralis may be released and, if necessary, a portion of the lateralis tendon itself can be lengthened (with suture repair after a 1- to 3-cm lengthening) to effect quadriceps balance.[105] This may be necessary in some cases of severe lateral pull with subluxation/dislocation in active extension and especially in congenital and obligatory dislocations associated with contracture of the vastus lateralis.[106,107]

The MPFL provides the primary soft-tissue static resistance to lateral displacement of the patella in flexion angles up to 30°. This ligament lies within the second, intermediate fascial layer and has attachments to the proximal half of the medial boarder of the patella and to an area just posterior to the medial femoral epicondyle in a sulcus lying between the adductor tubercle and the medial epicondyle. Most injuries to the MPFL during patellar dislocation occur at or near the femoral attachment; therefore, most often the native MPFL should be plicated or retensioned at its femoral attachment rather than its medial patellar border attachment. With acute patellar dislocation, injury to the MPFL and the need for repair is on the femoral side in about 90% of patients.[104]

In the treatment of chronic patellar instability, I generally prefer to isolate the retinacular layer inclusive of the MPFL, detach it from the tendon of the VMO, and then imbricate along the medial patellar border (Fig. 1). The existing retinacular tissue is far more forgiving of the undulating topography of the medial femoral condyle during flexion and extension and is more similar to the architecture of the native MPFL than is a rope-like hamstring tendon. The posteromedial corner of the tendon of the VMO is then advanced distally and posteriorly over the retensioned MPFL. The influence of the MPFL is greatest when the quadriceps are contracted with the knee in full extension, but strain measurements of the MPFL have shown the largest strain to be variable from 15° to 45° of flexion.[104] Therefore, I retension the MPFL with the knee at 30° of flexion with the patella centered

FIGURE 1

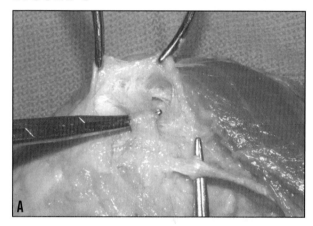

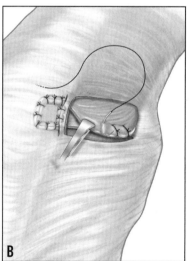

A, In this cadaver dissection, the intermediate layer of the medial retinaculum is isolated and mobilized from the capsule and then imbricated over the medial border of the patella. **B,** The tendon of the VMO is then advanced distally, with special care taken to secure the posteromedial corner.

within the trochlea as an estimate of maximal required length of the MPFL. The role of the MPFL is only to help guide the patella into the trochlea during the initial stages of knee flexion; it is not designed to have the primary responsibility of holding the patella in place once engaged within the trochlea. If this were so, the retinacular tissue would most certainly eventually stretch and fail.

MPFL reconstruction is most helpful for patients with recurrent patellar dislocations associated with hyperelasticity and for patients with obligatory patellar dislocations. Both of these scenarios are associated with incompetent medial retinacular tissue. I prefer the use of a semitendinosis autograft, and I follow techniques described by Avikainen and associates,[108] Deie and associates,[109] Gomes,[110] Muneta and associates,[111] and by Nomura and Inoue.[112] Others prefer to include MPFL reconstruction for patellar instability found in association with trochlear dysplasia.

After the medial side has been retensioned or reconstructed, the lateral retinaculum is repaired/lengthened as described by Larson and associates.[102] If a lateral retinacular release from previous surgery prevents adequate repair, then a transfer of the iliotibial band addresses reconstruction of the deep transverse lateral retinaculum. Hughston and associates[113] described a method of reconstruction for the lateral patellofemoral ligament using a distally based iliotibial band transfer. I prefer a proximally based transfer of the iliotibial band using the anterior 1 to 1.5 cm and suturing it to the proximal third of the lateral border of the patella (Fig. 2). As with reconstruction of the MPFL, I prefer to tension the lateral reconstruction with the patella engaged within the trochlea as the knee is

flexed 30°. The transfer originates at the level of the lateral femoral epicondyle, approximating the orientation of the native deep transverse retinacular ligament.

Patella alta is a common pathoanatomy associated with patellar dislocation, and inability to correct this deformity is a leading cause of failure of surgical stabilization.[54,114] Osteotomy of the tibial tuberosity with distal advancement has support within the literature.[115] Soft-tissue imbrication of the patellar tendon is less well understood, but has been used in my institution for patella alta associated with cerebral palsy. It has been considered but not validated for recurrent patellar dislocations.

When pathoanatomies include variances of trochlear shape or tuberosity position, osteotomy may be necessary. For malalignment resulting in an increased Q angle that is the result of an increased tibial tuberosity:trochlear groove distance, the Trillat method of tibial tuberosity transfer is reliable, stable, and effective.[116,117] If there are degenerative changes on the patella that are primarily on the lateral facet and/or mid or distal on the patella and if chronic anterior knee pain is present in addition to the recurrent patellar dislocations, then the anteromedial transfer of the tibial tuberosity as described by Fulkerson accomplishes both realignment as well as some degree of patellofemoral unloading.[40,118-120] If the abnormal Q angle is the result of excessive knee valgus, a distal femoral varus osteotomy may be a useful and necessary adjunct to the patellar realignment surgery.

Although trochlear dysplasia is one of the most common pathoanatomies associated with recurrent patellar dislocations, very little has been written regarding its sur-

FIGURE 2

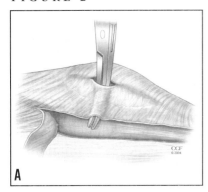 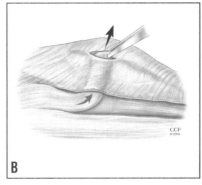 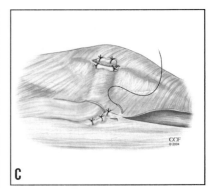

A, An interval is developed between the superficial oblique retinaculum and the underlying capsule. The deep transverse retinaculum is deficient from prior retinacular release. A 1- to 1.5-cm-wide strip of iliotibial tract is isolated and detached from Gerdy's tubercle and reflected proximally.
B, The isolated section of iliotibial tract is then redirected beneath the mobilized superficial oblique retinaculum to the lateral border of the patella.
C, With the knee flexed 30°, the transferred iliotibial tract is tensioned by progressively suturing distally to a level approximating the lateral femoral epicondyle. *(Reproduced with permission from the Campbell Clinic Foundation, Memphis, TN.)*

gical treatment.[52,121] Trochlear osteotomies are both difficult to perform and unproved as to long-term outcomes. The method of creating a sulcus by gouge or chisel has been reported.[122] As with any trochlear osteotomy, the effect on patellofemoral congruence is problematic and unresolved as to long-term importance.[123] The Albee osteotomy was first described in 1915 and then ignored in the literature until 1997.[124,125] I prefer this osteotomy for the trochlea with a hypoplastic lateral femoral condyle and a persistent lateral pull despite soft-tissue adjustments. It can be modified from the original descriptions, however, to become more anatomic and less disruptive of the articular cartilage. Original descriptions included 1 cm or more of elevation with bone grafting and fixation, but the normal trochlear sulcus is only 6 to 7 mm in depth. Therefore, elevation needs only to be performed with a 6- to 8-mm bone wedge. Furthermore, if the shape of the bone graft wedge is trapezoidal rather than rectangular, the anterior articular surface is less likely to be disrupted. I obtain the bone graft from the adjacent lateral femoral metaphysis. No internal fixation is required (Fig. 3). For a severely dysplastic trochlea that is convex and has a trochlear bump, the osteotomy described by Dejour is effective.[52,126] It requires a high level of planning and experience and should not be performed by anyone other than an experienced patellofemoral surgeon with special expertise in trochlear dysplasia.

The use of derotation osteotomy for the treatment of patellar instability remains controversial.[25,99] It is beyond the scope of this chapter to describe the details of indications, patient selection, and treatment outcomes for this procedure. That said, in some patients with internal femoral torsion or external tibial torsion or both as the primary pathoanatomy, the most appropriate treatment is derotation osteotomy. Caution should be maintained, however, because the surgery carries significant risks, and the mere existence of the deformity does not guarantee that correction of the deformity will result in a successful outcome.

MINIMALLY INVASIVE PATELLAR REALIGNMENT

Minimally invasive surgical techniques for patellar instability have been described.[127,128] They include a lateral retinacular release and a plication of the medial retinaculum. The plication may be performed with thermal wands or with percutaneous suture. The descriptions suggest selective plication of the MPFL, but the accuracy

FIGURE 3

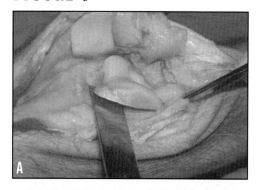
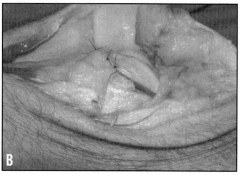

A, With the knee in extension, an osteotomy is performed from the trochlear entrance proximally to a point just anterior to the tibiofemoral articulation. *(Reproduced with permission from Andrish J, Valdevit R, Kuroda R, et al: Knee osteotomies and meniscal replacement effects on dynamic intra-joint loading. J Bone Joint Surg Am 2001;83:142-150.)* **B,** Careful elevation of the lateral femoral condyle 6 to 8 mm and insertion of a trapezoidal shaped autograft avoids articular cartilage disruption and restores trochlear depth.

of these techniques may be questioned. Short-term successes are reported, but long-term outcomes are needed. Morbidity and recovery are improved dramatically with a minimally invasive procedure compared to open realignments, but their ability to address the pathoanatomies of recurrent patellar dislocation is limited. Further testing is needed to determine whether the open approach of correcting the pathoanatomies of patellar instability results in superior long-term outcomes when compared with minimally invasive techniques. Intuition suggests that minimally invasive techniques will be helpful for the patient with patellar subluxations but not for the patient with recurrent patellar dislocations.

POSTOPERATIVE MANAGEMENT

Postoperative management requires individualization according to the combination of surgical tools used and the needs and expectations of the patient. The use of crutches with protected weight bearing is required until osteotomies have healed. Range of motion is emphasized early, regardless of the surgical techniques used, to minimize the potential complication of patellar entrapment and arthrofibrosis. Principles of pelvifemoral rehabilitation are incorporated to regain neuromotor recovery and stability. Return to full activity is affected by many patient and treatment factors and may range from 6 weeks to 6 months.

Conclusions

Recurrent patellar dislocations occur as a result of the presence of one or more abnormalities of the soft-tissue restraints, patellofemoral geometry, patellofemoral alignment, lower extremity alignment, and gait. The identification of the pathoanatomies unique to the individual with recurrent patellar dislocations is obtained from a careful physical examination as well as radiographs, and CT and/or MRI. Once these pathoanatomies have been identified for the individual patient, a systematic approach to surgical realignment and the selection of the components of the surgical procedure is possible.

References

1. Cohen ZA, Henry JH, McCarthy DM, Mow VC, Ateshian GA: Computer simulations of patellofemoral joint surgery. *Am J Sports Med* 2003;31:87-98.

2. Fithian DC, Paxton EW, Cohen AB: Indications in the treatment of patellar instability. *J Knee Surg* 2004;17:47-56.

3. Fithian DC, Paxton EW, Stone ML, Silva P, Davis DK, Elias DA, White LM: Epidemiology and natural history of acute patellar dislocation. *Am J Sports Med* 2004;32:1114-1121.

4. Crosby EB, Insall J: Recurrent dislocation of the patella: Relation of treatment to osteoarthritis. *J Bone Joint Surg Am* 1976;58:9-13.

5. Grelsamer RP, Weinstein CH: Applied biomechanics of the patella. *Clin Orthop* 2001;389:9-14.

6. Andrish J: The biomechanics of patellofemoral stability. *J Knee Surg* 2004;17:35-39.

7. Conlan T, Garth WP, Lemons JE: Evaluation of the medial soft-tissue restraints of the extensor mechanism of the knee. *J Bone Joint Surg Am* 1993;75:682-693.

8. Desio SM, Burks RT, Bachus KN: Soft tissue restraints to lateral patellar translation in the human knee. *Am J Sports Med* 1998;26:59-65.

9. Hautamaa PV, Fithian DC, Kaufman KR, Daniel DM, Pohlmeyer AM: Medial soft tissue restraints in lateral patellar instability and repair. *Clin Orthop* 1998;349:174-182.

10. Nomura E, Horiuchi Y, Kihara M: Medial patellofemoral ligament restraint in lateral patellar translation and reconstruction. *Knee* 2000;7:121-127.

11. Fithian DC, Nomura E, Arendt E: Anatomy of patellar dislocation. *Oper Tech Sports Med* 2001;9:102-111.

12. Amis AA, Firer P, Mountney J, Senavongse W, Thomas NP: Anatomy and biomechanics of the medial patellofemoral ligament. *Knee* 2003;10:215-220.

13. Senavongse W, Farahmand F, Jones J, Andersen H, Bull AMJ, Amis AA: Quantitative measurement of patellofemoral joint stability: Force-displacement behavior of the human patella in vitro. *J Orthop Res* 2003;21:780-786.

14. Farahmand F, Tahmasbi MN, Amis AA: Lateral force: Displacement behaviour of the human patella and its variation with knee flexion. A biomechanical study in vitro. *J Biomech* 1998;31:1147-1152.

15. Heegaard J, Leyvraz PF, Van Kampen A, Rakotomanna L, Rubin PJ, Blankevoort L: Influence of soft structures on patellar three-dimensional tracking. *Clin Orthop* 1994;299:235-243.

16. Lee TQ, Yang BY, Sandusky MD, McMahon PJ: The effects of tibial rotation on the patellofemoral joint: Assessment of the changes in in situ strain in the peripatellar retinaculum and the patellofemoral contact pressures and areas. *J Rehabil Res Dev* 2001;38:463-469.

17. Ahmed AM, Duncan NA: Correlation of patellar tracking pattern with trochlear and retropatellar surface topographies. *J Biomech Eng* 2000;122:652-660.

18. Carrillon Y, Abidi H, Dejour D, Fantino O, Moyen B, Tran-Minh VA: Patellar instability: Assessment on MR images by measuring the lateral trochlear inclination. Initial experience. *Radiology* 2000;216:582-585.

19. Neptune RR, Wright IC, van den Bogert AJ: The influence of orthotic devices and vastus medialis strength and timing on patellofemoral loads during running. *Clin Biomech* 2000;15:611-618.

20. Raimondo RA, Ahmad CS, Blankevoort L, April EW, Grelsamer RP, Henry JH: Patellar stabilization: A quantitative evaluation of the vastus medialis obliquus muscle. *Orthopedics* 1998;21:791-795.

21. Sakai N, Luo ZP, Rand JA, An KN: The influence of weakness in the vastus medialis oblique muscle on the patellofemoral joint: An in vitro biomechanical study. *Clin Biomech* 2000;15:335-339.

22. Goh JCH, Lee PYC, Bose K: A cadaver study of the function of the oblique part of vastus medialis. *J Bone Joint Surg Br* 1995;77:225-231.

23. Livingston LA: The quadriceps angle: A review of the literature. *J Orthop Sports Phys Ther* 1998;28:105-109.

24. Mizuno Y, Kumagai M, Mattessich SM, Elias JJ, Ramrattan N, Cosgarea AJ, Chao EYS: Q-angle influences tibiofemoral and patellofemoral kinematics. *J Orthop Res* 2001;19:834-840.

25. Post WR, Teitge R, Amis A: Patellofemoral malalignment: Looking beyond the viewbox. *Clin Sports Med* 2002;21: 521-546.

26. Sanfridsson J, Arnbjornsson A, Friden T, Ryd L, Svahn G, Jonsson K: Femorotibial rotation and the Q-angle related to the dislocating patella. *Acta Radiol* 2001;42:218-224.

27. Buckley SL, Barrack RL, Alexander AH: The natural history of conservatively treated partial anterior cruciate ligament tears. *Am J Sports Med* 1989;17:221-225.

28. Daniel DM, Stone ML, Dobson BE, Fithian DC, Rossman DJ, Kenton KR: Fate of the ACL-injured patient: A prospective outcome study. *Am J Sports Med* 1994;22:632-644.

29. McDaniel WJ, Dameron TB: Untreated ruptures of the anterior cruciate ligament. *J Bone Joint Surg Am* 1980;62:696-704.

30. Noyes FR, Mooar PA, Matthews DS, Butler DL: The symptomatic anterior cruciate-deficient knee: Part I. The long-term functional disability in athletically active individuals. *J Bone Joint Surg Am* 1983;65:154-162.

31. Dye SF: Patellofemoral pain current concepts: An overview. *Sports Med Arthrop Rev* 2001;9:264-272.

32. Arendt EA, Fithian DC, Cohen E: Current concepts of lateral patella dislocation. *Clin Sports Med* 2002;21:499-519.

33. James SL, Bates BT, Osternig LR: Injuries to runners. *Am J Sports Med* 1978;6:40-50.

34. James SL: Running injuries to the knee. *J Am Acad Orthop Surg* 1995;3:309-318.

35. Hutchinson MR, Ireland ML: Knee injuries in female athletes. *Sports Med* 1995;19:288-302.

36. Zeller BL, McCrory JL, Kibler B, Uhl TL: Differences in kinematics and electromyographic activity between men and women during the single-legged squat. *Am J Sports Med* 2003;31:449-456.

37. Hughston JC, Deese M: Medial subluxation of the patella as a complication of lateral retinacular release. *Am J Sports Med* 1988;16:383-388.

38. Atkin DM, Fithian DC, Marangi KS, Stone ML, Dobson BE, Mendelsohn C: Characteristics of patients with primary acute lateral patellar dislocation and their recovery within the first 6 months of injury. *Am J Sports Med* 2000;28:472-479.

39. Kolowich PA, Paulos LE, Rosenberg TD, Farnsworth S: Lateral release of the patella: Indications and contraindications. *Am J Sports Med* 1990;18:359-365.

40. Post WR, Fulkerson JP: Distal realignment of the patellofemoral joint: Indications, effects, results and recommendations. *Orthop Clin North Am* 1992;23:631-643.

41. Fulkerson JP: Anterolateralization of the tibial tubercle. *Tech Orthop* 1997;12:165-169.

42. DeLee JC, Drez D: Etiology of injury to the foot and ankle, in Stevenson A (ed): *Orthopaedic Sports Medicine: Principles and Practice*, ed 2. Philadelphia, PA, Saunders, 2003, vol 2, pp 2224-2274.

43. Steiner ME: Hypermobility and knee injuries. *Phys Sports Med* 1987;15:159-165.

44. Fithian DC, Mishra DK, Balen PF, Stone ML, Daniel DM: Instrumented measurement of patellar mobility. *Am J Sports Med* 1995;23:607-615.

45. Skalley TC, Terry GC, Teitge RA: The quantitative measurement of normal passive medial and lateral patellar motion limits. *Am J Sports Med* 1993;21:728-732.

46. Tanner SM, Garth WP, Soileau R, Lemons JE: A modified test for patellar instability: The biomechanical basis. *Clin J Sports Med* 2003;13:327-338.

47. Teitge RA, Faerber W, Des Madryl P, Matelic T: Stress radiographs of the patellofemoral joint. *J Bone Joint Surg Am* 1996;78:193-203.

48. Nonweiler DE, DeLee JC: The diagnosis and treatment of medial subluxation of the patella after lateral retinacular release. *Am J Sports Med* 1994;22:680-686.

49. Dejour H, Walch G, Nove-Josserand L, Guier CH: Factors of patellar instability: An anatomic radiographic study. *Knee Surg Sports Traumatol Arthrosc* 1994;2:19-26.

50. Dupont JY, Guier CA: Comparison of three standard radiologic techniques for screening of patellar subluxations. *Clin Sports Med* 2002;21:389-401.

51. Kujala UM, Osterman K, Kormano M, Nelimarkka O, Hurme M, Taimela S: Patellofemoral relationships in recurrent patellar dislocation. *J Bone Joint Surg Br* 1989;71: 788-792.

52. Dejour H, Walch G, Neyret PH, Adeleine P: Dysplasia of the femoral trochlea. *Rev Chir Orthop Reparatrice Appar Mot* 1990;76:45-54.

53. Galland O, Walch G, Dejour H, Carret JP: An anatomical and radiological study of the femoropatellar articulation. *Surg Radiol Anat* 1990;12:119-125.

54. Lancourt JE, Cristini JA: Patella alta and patella infera: Their etiological role in patellar dislocation, chondromalacia, and apophysitis of the tibial tubercle. *J Bone Joint Surg Am* 1975;57:1112-1115.

55. Nove-Josserand L, Dejour D: Quadriceps dysplasia and patellar tilt in objective patellar instability. *Rev Chir Orthop Reparatrice Appar Mot* 1995;81:497-504.

56. Tsujimoto K, Kurosaka M, Yoshiya S, Mizuno K: Radiographic and computed tomographic analysis of the position of the tibial tubercle in recurrent dislocation and subluxation of the patella. *Am J Knee Surg* 2000;13:83-88.

57. Beasley LS, Vidal AF: Traumatic patellar dislocation in children and adolescents: Treatment update and literature review. *Curr Opin Pediatr* 2004;16:29-36.

58. Murray TF, Dupont JY, Fulkerson JP: Axial and lateral radiographs in evaluating patellofemoral malalignment. *Am J Sports Med* 1999;27:580-584.

59. Berg EE, Mason SL, Lucas MJ: Patellar height ratios: A comparison of four measurement methods. *Am J Sports Med* 1996;24:218-221.

60. Laurin CA, Dussault R, Levesque HP: The tangential x-ray investigation of the patellofemoral joint: X-ray technique,

diagnostic criteria and their interpretation. *Clin Orthop* 1979;144:16-26.

61. Merchant AC, Mercer RL, Jacobsen RH, Cool CR: Roentgenographic analysis of patellofemoral congruence. *J Bone Joint Surg Am* 1974;56:1391-1396.

62. Kobayashi T, Fujikawa K: Theoretical use of 3D CT to predict method of patella realignment. *Knee* 2003;10:135-138.

63. Staubli HU, Durrenmatt U, Porcellini B, Rauschning W: Anatomy and surface geometry of the patellofemoral joint in the axial plane. *J Bone Joint Surg B*r 1999;81:452-458.

64. von Eisenhart-Rothe R, Siebert M, Bringmann C, Vogl T, Englmeier KH, Graichen H: A new in vivo technique for determination of 3D kinematics and contact areas of the patellofemoral and tibio-femoral joint. *J Biomech* 2004;27: 927-934.

65. Hawkins RJ, Bell RH, Anisette G: Acute patellar dislocations: The natural history. *Am J Sports Med* 1986;14:117-120.

66. Tuxoe JI, Teir M, Winge S, Nielsen PL: A medial patellofemoral ligament: A dissection study. *Knee Surg Sports Traumatol Arthrosc* 2002;10:138-140.

67. Harilainen A, Myllynen P: Operative treatment in acute patellar dislocation: Radiological predisposing factors, diagnosis and results. *Am J Knee Surg* 1988;1:178-185.

68. Maenpaa H, Lehto MU: Patellar dislocation: The long-term results of nonoperative management in 100 patients. *Am J Sports Med* 1997;25:213-217.

69. Brown DE, Alexander AH, Lightman DM: The Elmslie-Trillat procedure: Evaluation in patellar dislocation and subluxation. *Am J Sports Med* 1984;12:104-109.

70. Fondren FB, Goldner JL, Bassett FH: Recurrent dislocation of the patella treated by the modified Roux-Goldthwait procedure. *J Bone Joint Surg Am* 1985;67:993-1005.

71. Letts RM, Davidson D, Beaule P: Semitendinosus tenodesis for repair of recurrent dislocation of the patella in children. *J Pediatr Orthop* 1999;19:742-747.

72. Madigan R, Wissinger HA, Donaldson WF: Preliminary experience with a method of quadricepsplasty in recurrent subluxation of the patella. *J Bone Joint Surg Am* 1975;57:600-607.

73. Myers P, Williams A, Dodds R, Bulow J: The three-in-one proximal and distal soft tissue patellar realignment procedure: Results and its place in the management of patellofemoral instability. *Am J Sports Med* 1999;27:575-579.

74. Wootton JR, Cross MR, Wood DG: Patellofemoral malalignment: A report of 68 cases treated by proximal and distal patellofemoral reconstruction. *Injury* 1990;21: 169-173.

75. Aglietti P, Buzzi R, De Biase P, Giron F: Surgical treatment of recurrent dislocation of the patella. *Clin Orthop* 1994;308: 8-17.

76. Fulkerson JP, Schutzer SF, Ramsby GR, Bernstein RA: Computerized tomography of the patellofemoral joint before and after lateral release or realignment. *Arthroscopy* 1987;3:19-24.

77. Nikku R, Nietosvaara Y, Kallio PE, Aalto K, Michelsson JE: Operative versus closed treatment of primary dislocation of the patella. *Acta Orthop Scand* 1997;68:419-423.

78. Powers JA: Natural history of recurrent dislocation of the patella. *Clin Orthop* 1976:119:281.

79. Arnbjornsson A, Eglund N, Rydling O, Stockerup R, Ryd L: The natural history of recurrent dislocation of the patella: Long-term results of conservative and operative treatment. *J Bone Joint Surg Br* 1992;74:140-142.

80. Hampson WGJ, Hill P: Late results of transfer of the tibial tubercle for recurrent dislocation of the patella. *J Bone Joint Surg Br* 1975;57:209-213.

81. Juliusson R, Markhede G: A modified Hauser procedure for recurrent dislocation of the patella: A long-term follow-up study with special reference to osteoarthritis. *Arch Orthop Trauma Surg* 1984;103:42-46.

82. Maenpaa H, Lehto MU: Patellofemoral osteoarthritis after patellar dislocation. *Clin Orthop* 1997;339:156-162.

83. Nakagawa K, Wada Y, Minamide M, Tsuchiya A, Moriya H: Deterioration of long-term clinical results after the Elmslie-Trillat procedure for dislocation of the patella. *J Bone Joint Surg Br* 2002;84:861-864.

84. Shellock FG: Effect of a patellar realignment brace on patients with patellar subluxation and dislocation: Evaluation with kinematic magnetic resonance imaging. *Am J Sports Med* 2000;28:131-133.

85. Kuroda R, Kambic H, Valdevit A, Andrish JT: Articular cartilage contact pressure after tibial tuberosity transfer. *Am J Sports Med* 2001;29:409-409.

86. Huberti HH, Hayes WC: Patellofemoral contact pressures: The influence of Q-angle and tendofemoral contact. *J Bone Joint Surg Am* 1984;66:715-724.

87. Ahmed AM, Burke DL, Hyder A: Force analysis of the patellar mechanism. *J Orthop Res* 1987;5:69-85.

88. Pidoriano AJ, Weinstein RN, Buuck Da, Fulkerson JP: Correlation of patellar articular lesions with results from anteromedial tibial tubercle transfer. *Am J Sports Med* 1997;25:533-537.

89. Wilk KE, Davies GJ, Mangine RE, Malone TR: Patellofemoral disorders: A classification system and clinical guidelines for nonoperative rehabilitation. *J Orthop Sports Phys Ther* 1998;28:307-322.

90. Steinkamp LA, Dillingham MF, Markel MD, Hill JA, Kaufman KR: Biomechanical considerations in patellofemoral joint rehabilitation. *Am J Sports Med* 1993;21:438-444.

91. Farahmand F, Senavongse W, Amis A: Quantitative study of the quadriceps muscles and trochlear groove geometry related to instability of the patellofemoral joint. *J Orthop Res* 1998;16:136-143.

92. Grabiner MD, Koh TJ, Miller GF: Fatigue rates of vastus medialis oblique and vastus lateralis during static and dynamic knee extension. *J Orthop Res* 1991;9:391-397.

93. Lieb FJ, Perry J: Quadriceps function: An anatomical and mechanical study using amputated limbs. *J Bone Joint Surg Am* 1968;50:1535-1548.

94. Muhle C, Brinkmann G, Skaf A, Heller M, Resnick D: Effect of a patellar realignment brace on patients with patellar subluxation and dislocation. *Am J Sports Med* 1999;27:350-353.

95. Palumbo PM: Dynamic patellar brace: A new orthosis in the management of patellofemoral disorders. *Am J Sports Med* 1981;9:45-49.

96. Shellock FG: Effect of a patella-stabilizing brace on lateral subluxation of the patella. *Am J Knee Surg* 2000;13:137-142.

97. Harilainen A, Sandelin J: Prospective long-term results of operative treatment in primary dislocation of the patella. *Am Surg Sports Traumatol Arthrosc* 1993;1:100-103.

98. Godde S, Rupp S, Dienst M, Seil R, Kohn D: Fracture of the proximal tibia six months after Fulkerson osteotomy. *J Bone Joint Surg Br* 2001;83:832-833.

99. Teitge RA: Treatment of complications of patellofemoral joint surgery. *Oper Tech Sports Med* 1994;2:317-334.

100. Luo ZP, Sakai N, Rand JA, An KN: Tensile stress of the lateral patellofemoral ligament during knee motion. *Am J Knee Surg* 1997;10:139-144.

101. Ahmad CS, Sinicropi SM, Su B, Puffinbarger WF: Congenital medial dislocation of the patella. *Orthopedics* 2003;26:189-190.

102. Larson RL, Cabaud HE, Slocum DB, James SL, Kieenan T, Hutchinson T: The patellar compression syndrome: Surgical treatment by lateral retinacular release. *Clin Orthop* 1978;134:158-167.

103. Johnson DP, Wakeley C: Reconstruction of the lateral patellar retinaculum following lateral release: A case report. *Knee Surg Sports Traumatol Arthrosc* 2002;10:361-363.

104. Ahmad CS, Stein BES, Matuz D, Henry JH: Immediate surgical repair of the medial patellar stabilizers for acute patellar dislocation: A review of eight cases. *Am J Sports Med* 2000;22:804-810.

105. Hughston JC: Reconstruction of the extensor mechanism for subluxating patella. *J Sports Med* 1972;1:6-13.

106. Eilert RE: Dysplasia of the patellofemoral joint in children. *Am J Knee Surg* 1999;12:114-119.

107. Lai KA, Shen WJ, Lin CJ, Lin YT, Chen CY, Chang KC: Vastus lateralis fibrosis in habitual patella dislocation. *Acta Orthop Scand* 2000;71:394-398.

108. Avikainen VJ, Nikku RK, Seppanen-Lehmonen TK: Adductor magnus tenodesis for patellar dislocation. *Clin Orthop* 1993;297:12-16.

109. Deie M, Ochi M, Sumen Y, Yasumoto M, Kobayashi K, Kimura H: Reconstruction of the medial patellofemoral ligament for the treatment of habitual or recurrent dislocation of the patella in children. *J Bone Joint Surg Br* 2003;85:887-890.

110. Gomes JLE: Medial patellofemoral ligament reconstructino for recurrent dislocation of the patella: A preliminary report. *Arthroscopy* 1992;8:335-340.

111. Muneta T, Sekiya I, Tsuchiya M, Shinomiya K: A technique for reconstruction of the medial patellofemoral ligament. *Clin Orthop* 1999;359:151-155.

112. Nomura E, Inoue M: Surgical technique and rationale for medial patellofemoral ligament reconstruction for recurrent patellar dislocation. *Arthroscopy* 2003;19:1-9.

113. Hughston JC, Flandry F, Brinker MR, Terry GC, Mills JC: Surgical correction of medial subluxation of the patella. *Am J Sports Med* 1996;24:486-491.

114. Neyret Ph, Robinson AHN, LeCoultre B, Lapra C, Chambat P: Patellar tendon length: The factor in patellar instability? *Knee* 2002;9:3-6.

115. Simmons E Jr, Cameron JC: Patella alta and recurrent dislocation of the patella. *Clin Orthop* 1992;274:265-269.

116. Andrish JT: The Elmslie-Trillat Procedure. *Tech Orthop* 1997;12:1-8.

117. Kumar A, Jones S, Bickerstaff DR, Smith TWD: Functional evaluation of the modified Elmslie–Trillat procedure for patello-femoral dysfunction. *Knee* 2001;8:287-292.

118. Fulkerson JP, Becker GJ, Meaney JA, Miranda M, Folcik MA: Anteromedial tibial tubercle transfer without bone graft. *Am J Sports Med* 1990;18:490-497.

119. Nomura E, Inoue M: Cartilage lesions of the patella in recurrent patellar dislocation. *Am J Sports Med* 2004;32:498-502.

120. Post WR: Open patellar realignment for patellar pain and instability. *Oper Tech Sports Med* 1994;2:297-302.

121. Peterson L, Karlsson J, Brittberg M: Patellar instability with recurrent dislocation due to patellofemoral dysplasia results after surgical treatment. *Bull Hosp Jt Dis Orthop Inst* 1988;48:130-139.

122. Slocum B, Slocum TD: Trochlear wedge recession for medial patellar luxation. *Vet Clin North Am Small Anim Pract* 1993;23:869-875.

123. Kuroda R, Kambic H, Valdevit A, Andrish JT: Distribution of patellofemoral joint pressures after femoral trochlear osteotomy. *Knee Surg Sports Traumatol Arthrosc* 2002;10:33-37.

124. Albee FH: The bone graft wedge in the treatment of habitual dislocation of the patella. *Med Rec* 1915;88:257-259.

125. Weiker GT, Black KP: The anterior femoral osteotomy for patellofemoral instability. *Am J Knee Surg* 1997;10:221-227.

126. Masse Y: Trochleoplasty: Restoration of the intercondylar groove in subluxations and dislocations of the patella. *Rev Chir Orthop Reparatrice Appar Mot* 1978;64:3-17.

127. Haspl M, Cicak N, Klobucar H, Pecina M: Fully arthroscopic stabilization of the patella. *Arthroscopy* 2002;18:1-3.

128. Small NC, Glogau AI, Berezin MA: Arthroscopically assisted proximal extensor mechanism realignment of the knee. *Arthroscopy* 1993;9:63-67.

CHAPTER 7

PATELLOFEMORAL ARTHRITIS WITH MALALIGNMENT

ANTHONY A. SCHEPSIS, MD

FREDERICK J. WATSON, MD

Anterior knee pain secondary to chondrosis or arthrosis of the patellofemoral articulation is often difficult to manage. Patients often have associated patellar malalignment and/or instability. The etiology of patellofemoral pain is multifactorial; therefore, other causes of anterior knee pain must be ruled out before attributing the pain to lesions of the articular cartilage in the patellofemoral articulation. This chapter discusses the use of tibial tubercle transfer in patients with patellofemoral arthrosis with malalignment and/or instability, the decision-making process used in assessing malalignment of the patellofemoral articulation, the criteria for tibial tubercle transfer in both the medial and anteromedial direction, and surgical techniques.

According to the classification of Fulkerson,[1] malalignment is defined as an abnormal tilt and/or subluxation of the patella. Axial and lateral radiographs of the patellofemoral joint, such as the Merchant or Laurin view (Fig. 1), or CT may be used to assess lateral tilt and subluxation of the patella in reference to the trochlea.[2-8] When discussing tibial tubercle osteotomies or distal realignments, however, the term malalignment is used more specifically in reference to the tibial tubercle being in a more lateral position than what is considered to be normal. Unfortunately, there is no wide agreement on what is considered normal because the position of the tibial tubercle relative to the trochlear sulcus varies widely. Furthermore, it cannot be assumed that a patient with a clinical examination and radiographic and CT findings consistent with tibial tubercle malalignment has pain and arthrosis secondary to this factor because many such individuals are asymptomatic. Careful evaluation of all possible etiologies must be explored before attributing patellofemoral pain to malalignment.

BONY CONSIDERATIONS AND TUBERCLE MALALIGNMENT

The medial patellofemoral ligament provides soft-tissue stability to the patellofemoral joint. The soft tissues are primarily responsible for the stability of the patella in the trochlea in the first 30° of flexion, whereas the bony anatomy becomes more critical beyond 30° of flexion.

FIGURE 1

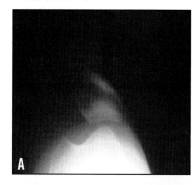
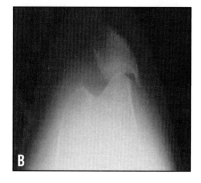

Axial radiographs of the knee. **A,** 30° axial view demonstrating patellar tilt and subluxation. **B,** 30° axial view demonstrating marked tilt, subluxation, and arthrosis of the lateral facet.

Overall limb alignment should be considered when evaluating patellofemoral malalignment. Although the tibial tubercle may be in a lateral position relative to the trochlear sulcus, this anatomic entity may more likely come from torsional abnormalities, particularly internal femoral torsion and external tibial torsion. Foot malalignment, particularly foot pronation, should be corrected orthotically if present. Valgus alignment of the extremity also places the tubercle in a relatively lateral position and predisposes it to malalignment.

It is very important to recognize the presence or absence of bony dysplasia of the trochlea and/or patella. In particular, trochlear dysplasia, reported on by Dejour and associates,[9] may lead to patellar instability, malalignment, and subsequent arthrosis with progressive insufficiency of the medial patellofemoral ligament. True lateral radiographs may reveal dysplasia, often associated with a trochlear "bump." Teitge (R Teitge, MD, San Diego, CA, unpublished data, 2003) described the reconstruction of the medial patellofemoral ligament in patients with trochlear dysplasia. Trochleoplasty has been used in Europe to deepen the trochlear groove in severe cases of trochlear dysplasia, but this difficult procedure is less commonly used in the United States, and there are many concerns regarding complications, particularly violation of the articular surface.

Basic to the surgical treatment of patellar malalignment with arthrosis is the process of moving the tibial tubercle in a medial or anteromedial direction; therefore, it is important to understand the methods of measuring tubercle malalignment, or lateralization of the tibial tubercle. A number of clinical and radiographic methods are available to measure tubercle alignment and position. The most common measure is the quadriceps angle, or Q angle, which measures the angle between a line drawn from the anterior superior iliac spine to the midpoint of the patella and a line drawn from the midportion of the patella to the midpoint of the tibial tubercle (Fig. 2). A Q angle greater than 15° in women or 12° in men is generally considered abnormal; however, this criterion is somewhat arbitrary. In the literature, the Q angle is variously described and measured with the patient in the standing, sitting, and supine positions, and with the knee in various degrees of flexion. We believe that the most accurate Q angle measurement is made with the knee at 30° of flexion, because the patella should be well centered in the trochlear groove by 20° to 25° of flexion. We recommend, however, that the Q angle be measured at various degrees of flexion to adequately show how the patella tracks in the groove. We also measure the Q angle with the knee in extension as well as at greater degrees of flexion. It is important to recognize J-tracking, which is defined as the abrupt shift of the patella laterally when the knee reaches terminal extension. J-tracking indicates a valgus vector force on the patella secondary to relative lateral tubercle malalignment. Measurement of the Q angle

FIGURE 2

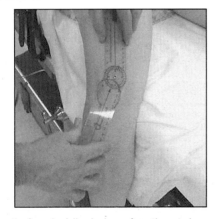

Measuring the Q angle. A line is drawn from the anterior superior iliac spine to the center of the patella, and a second line is drawn from the center of the patella to the center of the tibial tubercle. The angle between the two is the Q angle.

FIGURE 3

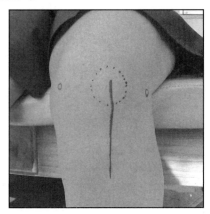

The tuberosulcus angle is the angle between a line drawn perpendicular to the transepicondylar axis and a line drawn from the midpoint of the patella to the tubercle. Measured with the knee at 90° of flexion, this is another measure of tubercle malalignment.

with the knee in full extension in these patients will result in a falsely low value because the patella is in a lateral position.

The tuberosulcus angle, which represents the angle between a line drawn perpendicular to the transepicondylar axis and a line drawn from the midpoint of the patella to the tubercle, is measured with the patient in a sitting position and the knee in 90° of flexion (Fig. 3). The angle normally measures 0°; a tuberosulcus angle greater than 10° is considered abnormal.[10]

CT is standard protocol in our practice to assess patellar tracking and instability and to calculate tibial tubercle malalignment. To assess patellar tracking, we first obtain a set of tracking images, which are mid-axial CT cuts through the patellofemoral joint at the midpoint of the patella from 0° to 60° in 10° increments (Fig. 4). This allows tracking measurements in early flexion, where instability usually occurs, and produces more precise anatomic measurements of the lateral patellofemoral angle to denote tilt and congruence angle to detect subluxation.

The second set of images we obtain consists of axial cuts from just above the trochlear groove distally through the tibial tuberosity. The radiographic Q angle or the anterior tibial tubercle-trochlear groove (ATT-TG) distance can be measured on this set of images (Fig. 5). The ATT-TG distance is a CT measurement of the distance between the center of the trochlear groove and the center of the attachment of the patellar tendon on the tibial tubercle. An ATT-TG distance greater than 2 cm is considered highly abnormal, representing excessive lateralization of the tibial tubercle with a high valgus vector on the knee. Although studies suggest that the normal range is 2 to 9 mm and greater than 10 mm is abnormal,[5,11] the exact cut-off between "normal" and "abnormal" is very difficult to ascertain because of the very wide range of anatomic variations.

PROCEDURE SELECTION

Most cases of recurrent lateral patellar instability are multifactorial, thus requiring careful evaluation when choosing the best surgical option. For example, in a young patient with traumatic onset of lateral patellar instability

FIGURE 4

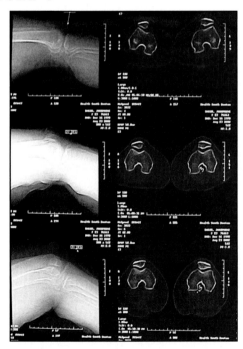

Patellofemoral tracking study. Axial CT images through the midpoint of the patella are taken at 10° increments from 0° to 60° of flexion. In this case, J-tracking is demonstrated as the patella is subluxated and tilted in extension (top row of images) and quickly becomes congruent in early flexion (bottom 2 rows).

FIGURE 5

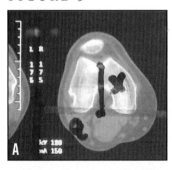

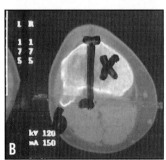

Measure of the ATT-TG distance. Axial images are taken from the proximal trochlea through the tibial tubercle on the same sequence with the extremity fixed in extension. **A,** A line is drawn along the posterior femoral condyles on the cut through the deepest portion of the trochlear groove. A perpendicular (x) is drawn from the center of the groove to this line and measured. The distance (a) is measured from this intersection to a fixed point, in this case, the edge of the frame. **B,** The same parallel line is transposed with a parallel rule to the cut through the midportion of the tendon attachment on the tubercle at the same perpendicular distance (x). The distance (b) is measured to the same fixed point. The ATT-TG distance is a–b. In this instance, it was 5 mm, well within normal range.

secondary to a patellar dislocation, recurrent episodes, abnormal lateral patellar glide, and relatively normal clinical and radiographic alignment, the most likely diagnosis is insufficiency of the medial patellofemoral ligament. Treatment should consist of a proximal realignment with attention to the medial patellofemoral ligament. Conversely, for a patient who has a markedly abnormal Q angle with minimally increased lateral patellar glide with radiographic tilt and subluxation, a distal realignment procedure is a better choice.

Unfortunately, because of the multifactorial nature of this problem, most cases are not quite that simple and the etiology of occurrence (traumatic versus atraumatic) as well as anatomic and biomechanical factors must be considered. In general, a traumatic onset is more likely to be associated with damage to the proximal and medial soft-tissue restraints, whereas an atraumatic onset is more likely to be associated with a malalignment problem. Furthermore, the status of the articular cartilage is very important. There are concerns that a proximal medial imbrication or reconstruction of the medial patellofemoral ligament potentially tethers the medial facet and increases contact pressures in this area (A Lehman, MD, et al, Phoenix, AZ, unpublished data, 2003). On the other hand, tubercle transfer in a medial direction will also transfer forces to the medial facet but not tether the facet and increase contact pressures.

HISTORY AND PHYSICAL EXAMINATION

The complete evaluation of a patient with anterior knee pain is discussed in chapter 3. The focus here is the patient with patellar instability and/or malalignment associated with related cartilage breakdown, which is thought to be the primary cause of the patient's patellofemoral symptoms. Although the patient presents with symptoms of patellofemoral arthrosis, the condition may be secondary to the underlying malalignment, causing abnormal contact pressures across the patellofemoral joint. The history should determine whether the patient has symptomatic instability, either subluxation or dislocation, or purely patellofemoral pain secondary to chondrosis or arthrosis associated with the malalignment.

Physical examination of a patient with symptomatic chondrosis or arthrosis should include determining the flexion arc in which the patient has pain. This finding is sometimes a clue as to the location of the disease. Pain in the terminal arc of extension or early range of flexion and crepitus indicate a more distal lesion, a painful arc and crepitus between 30° and 70° indicates a midpatellar lesion, and painful crepitus in higher degrees of flexion indicates a more proximal lesion on the patella. Accurate localization of the patellar lesion is very important in determining whether or not an anterior or medial transfer is indicated. The integrity of the medial patellofemoral ligament is assessed by measuring the amount of lateral patellar glide at 30° and comparing it with the contralateral knee. Careful palpation of the facets circumferentially can be helpful. Assessing passive patellar tilt to determine tightness of the lateral retinaculum is important in helping to decide whether a lateral retinacular release is necessary.

DISTAL REALIGNMENT BY MEDIAL TIBIAL TUBERCLE TRANSFER

Our principal indications for medial tibial tubercle transfer include (1) lateral patellar instability and/or patellar malalignment with moderate to severe static malalignment with radiographic or CT evidence of tilt and/or subluxation; (2) tubercle malalignment with normal or only mild insufficiency of the medial patellofemoral ligament; (3) lateral patellar instability associated with patella alta; (4) a patella with a J-tracking patern; and (5) advanced medial arthrosis that causes concern about tethering the medial facet by proximal realignment.

Tightening the proximal medial restraints in the presence of significant patella alta creates abnormal forces and does not correct the problem. In these patients, the patella centers into the groove in higher degrees of flexion. Some of the best results of distal realignment or medial tubercle transfers are in patients with patella alta and lateral patellar instability. Likewise, J-tracking, where the patella "jumps" out laterally in terminal extension, is an indicator of a valgus vector from bony malalignment, which starts at the hip from internal femoral torsion. The more practical solution is to make the correction at the tibial tubercle, although on a theoretical basis, a femoral derotation osteotomy would correct the problem at its source.

Distal realignment offers the following advantages: (1) it addresses one of the more common predisposing factors, tubercle malalignment; (2) it allows an aggressive rehabilitation program; (3) patients are less likely to have problems with range of motion than are patients who undergo open proximal reconstructions or imbrications; (4) the risk of tethering the medial facet of the patella with an overconstrained proximal realignment is less, even though pressure transfers go from lateral to medial on the patella when transposing the tubercle medially; (5) the procedure involves less violation of the extensor mechanism than proximal procedures; and (6) medial tubercle transfer corrects lateral subluxation (congruence angle) as well as lateral patellar tilt (lateral patellofemoral angle).

Numerous authors have reviewed the effects of medialization and anteromedialization on patellofemoral mechanics. The effect of anterior displacement of the tuberosity on patellofemoral contact forces is discussed later; however, many studies have shown that medial tubercle transfer corrects tilt as well as subluxation and transfers force from the patellofemoral joint from a lateral to a medial direction.[8,12-27]

Gill and associates (T Gill, MD, et al, San Diego, CA, unpublished data, 2003) reported that increasing the Q angle increases patellofemoral contact pressures and transfers forces to the lateral facet of the patella as well as tilts and subluxates the patella laterally. They also demonstrated that medialization corrects the maltracking and partially corrects the increased contact pressures in the patellofemoral articulation.

Medial tubercle transfer, however, is contraindicated in patients with a normal Q angle or no clinical or radiographic evidence of tubercle malalignment. In a cadaver study, Kuroda and associates[28] found that medialization in the presence of a normal Q angle increased patellofemoral contact pressures and increased the contact pressures in the medial tibiofemoral compartment. They concluded that overmedialization should be avoided in the varus knee, the knee with medial compartment arthrosis, or the knee with previous total or subtotal medial meniscectomy.

Distal realignment is sometimes indicated in combination with proximal realignment when there is both traumatic insufficiency of the medial patellofemoral ligament and tubercle malalignment. In these cases, both abnormalities need to be corrected.

The disadvantages of distal realignment, which should be recognized before performing this procedure, include: (1) the procedure does not address an incompetent medial patellofemoral ligament; (2) it cannot be performed properly before skeletal maturity; (3) it requires internal fixation, which often needs to be removed; (4) posterior neurovascular complications are possible when using an anterior to posteriorly directed bicortical screw in the proximal tibia; (5) osseous delayed or nonunion is possible; and (6) increased loading of the medial tibiofemoral compartment occurs, contraindicating the use of the procedure in the varus knee or knee with medial compartment arthrosis.

Technique of Medial Tibial Tubercle Transfer

Medial tibial tubercle transfer was first described by Trillat and associates[29] in 1964 and then popularized by Cox[15] as the Elmslie-Trillat procedure. Before beginning the procedure, arthroscopy is performed to address any associated lesions, followed by chondroplasty if necessary, and patellar tracking is assessed. At this time, a decision must be made whether to perform anteromedialization or straight medialization. In general, even if arthroscopy reveals significant chondral changes, straight medialization to correct patellar instability and/or malalignment is indicated if the patient is not symptomatic of the chondrosis or arthrosis. If the patient has symptomatic arthrosis or chondrosis, the location and severity of the lesion should be noted before deciding which direction to move the tibial tubercle. In some patients with very severe generalized grade IV disease of both the patella and trochlea, no further surgery may be indicated at this time, and the patient may be a better candidate for other procedures.

The next decision is whether or not to perform a lateral retinacular release, either arthroscopic or open. Lateral retinacular release is performed when there is either excessive tightness of the lateral retinaculum secondary to a negative passive patellar tilt, symptomatic arthrosis or chondrosis in the lateral compartment of the patellofemoral joint, or radiographic or CT imaging evidence of a decreased lateral patellofemoral angle. Lateral release alone is indicated only for excessive lateral pressure syndrome, with lateral facet pain, a tight lateral retinaculum, minimal or only grade 1 or 2 lateral facet changes, and no subluxation or clinical instability symptoms.

The medial tibial tubercle transfer is performed through a 3- to 4-cm longitudinal incision just lateral to the tibial tubercle (Fig. 6, A). A 1- to 1.5-cm-thick, 5- to 6-cm-long osteoperiosteal shingle is created with hand osteotomes. The patellar tendon is mobilized so that the undersurface of its attachment can be well visualized with retraction (Fig. 6, B). The first cut is performed from lateral to medial with a 1- to 1.5-in-wide hand

FIGURE 6

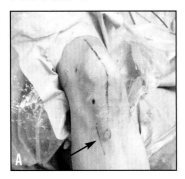

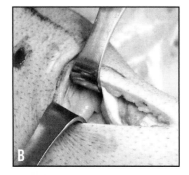

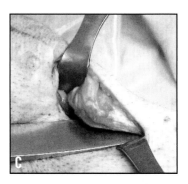

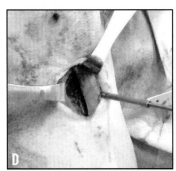

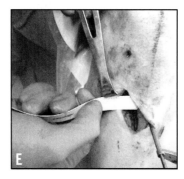

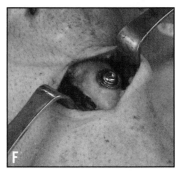

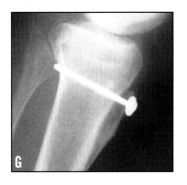

Tibial tubercle medialization (Elmslie-Trillat procedure). **A,** Lateral incision is indicated by the arrow. **B,** Exposing the patellar tendon. Both sides of the tendon must be freed up to prevent tethering when the tubercle is shifted. **C,** For medialization, a 1- to 1.5-cm-thick, 5- to 6-cm-long shingle is adequate. It is left attached by periosteum distally at the anterior cortex. The osteotomy is performed with hand osteotomes from lateral to medial. The osteotomy must be made exactly in the coronal plane for true medialization. Care must be taken not to angle posteriorly, or posteromedialization will occur, which could lead to overloading. **D,** The osteotomy is temporarily fixed and patellofemoral tracking assessed. **E,** The amount of medialization is measured. A 10- to 15-mm transfer is usually adequate. The Q angle should be corrected to less than 10°. **F,** The osteotomy is fixed with an 4.5-mm AO bicortical screw and washer. **G,** Lateral radiograph showing a completed tibial tubercle medialization.

osteotome 1-cm thick at the level of the tibial tubercle (Fig. 6, *C*). Care should be taken to make this osteotomy exactly in the coronal plane. It is best to err on the side of cutting from posterior to anterior when going from the lateral to the medial direction so that when the tubercle is transferred, it will move slightly anteriorly and never posteriorly, which would increase patellofemoral contact pressures. A mark is made on the skin 5 to 6 cm distal to the tubercle, and a curved osteotome is used to aim for this point to angle sharply toward the anterior cortex. A small osteotome is used to complete the osteotomy transversely just on the proximal side of the tibial tubercle to prevent propagation into the tibial plateau. Osteoclasis is performed, leaving the distal soft tissues intact, and the tibial tubercle is gently rotated medially. The parameters we use are that the patella is fully engaged and congruent by 20° of flexion and the Q angle is corrected to less than 10° as measured intraoperatively with a large sterile metal goniometer. Temporary fixation is achieved with a 3.2-mm AO drill bit inserted to, but not through, the posterior cortex, at which time a final assessment of tracking is made (Fig. 6, *D*). In general, the transfer ranges from a 1- to 1.5-cm shift, depending on the severity of the tubercle malalignment (Fig. 6, *E*). If the surgeon is satisfied with the degree of tubercle transfer and the tracking is satisfactory, fixation is performed with a fully threaded 4.5-mm bicortical screw with metal washer (Fig. 6, *F* and *G*). Because the shingle is short and thin, we routinely use only one bicortical screw, allowing rigid fixation and an aggressive postoperative rehabilitation program. For larger shingles, fixation with two screws may be considered. Care must be taken when drilling through the posterior cortex of the tibia in this area. The drilling should be performed with the knee in at least 90° of flexion, with care taken not to plunge through the posterior cortex. When medial patellofemoral ligament deficiency is a problem and instability and tracking are not fully corrected, these issues can be addressed either arthroscopically or with an open procedure at this time.

We use the tourniquet for the open part of the procedure and then release it before closure to achieve hemostasis. A drain is not usually necessary as it is for anteromedialization. The subcutaneous tissues and skin are closed carefully and the patient is placed in a long leg brace locked in extension.

Rehabilitation

Cosgarea and associates[14] reported on the biomechanics of flat versus oblique tibial tubercle osteotomy. In patients who undergo straight medial tubercle transfer with a small, thin, flat osteotomy, early weight bearing may be allowed, whereas a patient with an anteromedialized tubercle, with a larger oblique osteotomy, should delay weight bearing for the first 4 to 6 weeks after surgery.

In general, full range of motion is allowed immediately, and full range of motion is usually regained within a couple of weeks after surgery. Protected weight bearing for the first 3 to 4 weeks with the brace locked in extension is encouraged, until the patient has good quadriceps control. Because the quadriceps and extensor mechanism are not violated, early quadriceps isometrics are allowed, with resistive quadriceps strengthening allowed at 6 to 8 weeks, at which point some early bony healing has occurred.

Results

Several authors have reported a very high success rate for medial tibial tubercle transfer with a low rate of complications in large series of patients.[15,27,30] These clinical studies have reported the following conclusions: (1) the procedure is best used in young patients without evidence of severe systematic chondrosis or arthrosis; (2) medial tubercle transfer corrects subluxation (congruence angle) as well as tilt (lateral patellofemoral angle); (3) adequate postoperative Q angle correction (to < 10°) correlates with a good outcome; (4) patella alta patients do well with this procedure; and (5) screw removal is common.

COMBINED DISTAL AND PROXIMAL REALIGNMENT

A combination of distal and proximal realignment is indicated for tubercle malalignment and traumatic incompetency of the medial restraints, particularly the medial patellofemoral ligament. This combination of problems usually occurs in patients with recurrent (traumatic onset) lateral instability leading to proximal insufficiency, a static lateral position of the patella from distal malalignment, an increased Q angle, and radiographic evidence of tilt and/or subluxation. Our approach, which includes correction of the tubercle malalignment followed by reassessment of patellar tracking, eliminates the valgus vector pulling the patella laterally. If only proximal realignment is performed in these patients, the Q angle and the valgus vector forces are increased and create abnormal stresses on the patellofemoral joint. If patellar tracking and lateral instability of the patella remain a problem after the tubercle malalignment correction, we then perform the additional proximal realignment. In our practice, arthroscopic medial imbrication has sufficiently corrected the problem in most patients. Open reconstruction of the medial patellofemoral ligament, which is performed in cases of severe insufficiency, has been necessary only rarely.

SYMPTOMATIC ARTHROSIS AND ANTEROMEDIALIZATION

When pain is an important or the only symptom in combination with malalignment, a decision must be made whether to move the tubercle straight medially or anteromedially or whether a tubercle transfer should be avoided altogether. In general, anteriorization and medialization may be considered in patients with lateral or distal symptomatic chondrosis or arthrosis. Treatment algorithms for the decision of which direction the tibial tubercle should be transferred are shown in Table 1.

When considering tibial tubercle osteotomy for patellofemoral arthrosis with malalignment, it is important to define which patients will most benefit from anteromedialization. The most likely candidates are patients with pain secondary to symptomatic arthrosis of the patellofemoral articulation with malalignment, with or without symptoms of lateral patellar instability. The goal is to unload and relieve the pain of symptomatic lesions as well as to realign by anteriorization of the tibial tubercle. In

TABLE 1

Tibial Tubercle Transfer Direction

Tubercle Transfer Direction	Medial	Instability with malalignment: No arthrosis	
	Anteromedial	Malalignment with arthrosis	Malalignment > arthrosis, moderate obliquity
			Arthrosis > malalignment, maximum obliquity
	Anterior	Distal arthrosis with no malalignment (poor lateral restraints)	

accomplishing this, care must be to taken to avoid loading other areas of diseased cartilage and causing more pain.

Anteriorization of the tibial tubercle dates back to 1963 with the Maquet[31-34] principle, which may have actually first been described by Bandi[35] in 1972. The Maquet principle stated that elevation of the tibial tubercle reduces patellar tendon forces and decreases the vector angle between the quadriceps and the patellar tendon force, thus reducing the resultant patellofemoral joint reaction vector force. In Maquet's[31-34] initial biomechanical studies, he concluded that 2 cm of advancement of the tibial tubercle reduced the compressive patellar forces by about 50% and also decreased the tibiofemoral contact forces. According to his theory, the more the tubercle was elevated, the more the patellofemoral contact forces were decreased. In the 1970s and 1980s, in both Europe and the US, this procedure was commonly used for patients with symptomatic patellofemoral arthrosis. Unfortunately, elevation of the tibial tubercle up to 2 cm led to many complications, such as skin necrosis, wound breakdown, infection, fracture, and nonunion. Furthermore, Maquet did not account properly for rotational or horizontal vectors and he assumed incorrectly that the vector force of the quadriceps pull was equal to the vector force of the patellar tendon pull. Subsequently, between Ferguson and associates'[16] hallmark study in 1979 and the present, many authors have studied tibial tubercle transfer extensively.[16-21,23-26,36-54] A summary of some of these studies is shown in Table 2.

To summarize, biomechanical studies have shown the following: (1) Anteriorization of the tibial tubercle should not exceed 12 to 15 mm because further elevation has minimal biomechanical effect, it may have a deleterious effect by loading the proximal portion of the patella, as well as increasing the risk of complications. In particular, wound complications increase dramatically with elevation of more than 15 mm. (2) The procedure decreases contact pressures, mostly on the distal and lateral portions of the patella. (3) Anteriorization rotates the patella on its horizontal axis and relieves pressure in the distal portion of the patella; however, it loads the proximal portion of the patella. This finding is particularly evident at elevations of more than 15 mm. (4) Anteromedialization of the tibial tubercle shifts contact forces from the distal lateral portion of the patella to the proximal medial portion of the patella. (5) Anterior or anteromedial tibial tubercle transfer produces an extremely variable effect from patient to patient because every tracking pattern is different and the problem is multifactorial. There is a wide range of changes and shifting of contact pressures with anteromedialization and anteriorization.[8]

Clinical confirmation of these biomechanical findings has been further demonstrated by the excellent clinical studies by Fulkerson and associates.[19,38,45,46] They reported that the patients who benefited most from anteromedialization of the tibial tubercle were those with chrondrosis or arthrosis in the lateral or distal portion of the patella.

Fulkerson and associates[19,38] first described anteromedialization of the tibial tubercle in 1983, with a follow-up in 1990. This procedure is indicated for patients with patellar malalignment consisting of tilt and/or subluxation in association with arthrosis, preferably in the areas described. Their biomechanical studies were in concert with others showing that anteriorization of 12 to 15 mm and medialization of 9 to 10 mm of the tibial tubercle result in decreased lateral facet pressures and a shifting of the

contact pressures of the patella proximally and medially.[8,12,16-18,20,21,41]

To maximize anteriorization and minimize medialization in patients with arthrosis that is greater than mal-

TABLE 2

Results of Anteriorization Studies

Author	Study Design	Conclusions
Ferguson and associates[16]	Cadaver study. Elevations of 0.5, 1.0, and 1.5 in were evaluated at 0°, 45°, and 90°.	Tubercle elevation decreases stresses at all angles. Most pronounced at 90°. Minimal relief after 1.25-cm elevation.
Nakamura[21]	Cadaver study. Elevations of 1, 2, and 3 cm and length of split evaluated.	1-cm elevation optimal in reducing patellofemoral contact stresses. 2- and 3-cm elevation decreased congruity and size of contact area. Increased forces on proximal patella with higher elevation. The shorter the shingle, the greater the distal shift and rotation of the patella, increasing stresses on proximal pole.
Ferrandez and associates[18]	Cadaver study. Elevation of 0.5, 1.0, 1.5, 2.0, and 2.5 cm were evaluated	1-cm elevation most efficient. With higher elevations, although overall contact pressure decreases, zones of higher pressure are encountered more proximally ("tipping effect").
Fulkerson and associates[19]	Cadaver study. Anteromedialization with 8.8-mm anteriorization/8.4-mm medialization compared with 14.8 mm/8.4 mm.	Contact pressures reduced most significantly on lateral facet. Contact area moved slightly proximal with anteriorization.
Radin and Pan[26]	Tibial shingle length evaluated.	Short shingle causes excessive "tipping" of the proximal pole. Longer shingle minimizes this "tipping" effect.
Benevenuti and associates[12]	Simulations of 1.0-, 1.5-, and 2-cm elevations and 0.5 and 1 cm medializations on computer-generated models of cadaver knees.	Increasing tubercle elevation decreased lateral and medial peak pressure between 45° and 60° of knee flexion. At greater than 60° of flexion, however, increasing elevation decreased lateral pressures but increased medial pressures.
Cohen and associates[8]	Computer-generated models of 20 patients with patellofemoral symptoms. Simulations of anteriorization and anteromedialization performed.	Anteriorization and anteromedialization both reduced patellofemoral contact stresses on average, but results were patient specific. Must determine appropriate transfer on case-by-case basis.
Ramappa (unpublished data, 2003)	Cadaver study. Evaluated mechanics of increased Q angle, medialization, and anteromedialization.	Medialization and anteromedialization both decreased the increased contact pressures caused by an increased Q angle.

alignment, the obliquity of the cut may be varied so that maximal obliquity (which is limited by the lateral intermuscular septum to approximately 60°) is achieved. Conversely, when malalignment is the greater problem, an osteotomy with less obliquity may be created for more medialization. In summary, most biomechanical and clinical studies suggest that the location of the arthrois is a much more important factor than the extent of disease.

Indications for Anteromedialization

Anteromedialization is indicated as follows: (1) in patients with symptomatic arthrosis of the patellofemoral joint that is located in the lateral or distal portion of the patella associated with clinical and radiographic evidence of malalignment consisting of tilt and/or subluxation (Fig. 7); (2) following failure of an extensive nonsurgical rehabilitation program; and (3) in combination with cartilage restoration procedures of the patella or trochlea to unload and protect the concomitant procedures, unless the primary symptomatic and treated lesion is located on the proximal one third of the patella. These patients may have undergone a cartilage restoration procedure such as microfracture, autologous chondrocyte implantation, or a patellar or trochlear osteoarticular transfer system (mosiacplasty) procedure, and anteromedialization is often combined with these procedures to correct malalignment and unload the treated areas of the articular cartilage.

In most patients with symptomatic arthrosis (unless it is secondary to direct trauma), a degree of malalignment is present that may be subtle and can be identified only by the CT studies described earlier. Careful assessment of the tubercle alignment is mandatory.

Technique

Anteromedialization is performed through a laterally based incision (Fig. 8, *A*). If necessary, a lateral retinacular release is performed (Fig. 8, *B*). If there are preexisting incisions, a skin bridge of at least 5 cm is mandatory and the incision may be modified if necessary. It is important to free up the patellar tendon on both sides to allow proper transfer of shift in forces to the patella (Fig. 8, *C*). The tibialis anterior is carefully dissected subperiosteally off the lateral tibial crest, back to the limit of the lateral intermuscular septum. The osteotomy should be approximately 8 cm in length, so the incision should allow adequate exposure of the tibia for this purpose (Fig. 8, *D*).

We prefer to use an AMZ Guide (DePuy-Mitek, Norwood, MA) as developed in conjunction with Jack Farr, MD (Fig. 8, *E*). This is helpful to predetermine the exact obliquity of the cut, as well as to ensure a flat cut so that there are no incongruities in the contact areas between the two surfaces when shifting the tubercle anteriorly and medially. As an alternative, a flat pin block from a commercially available external fixation system can be used.

The AMZ Guide is placed in the proposed spot, and a specially designed caliper may be placed inside the holes of the guide to determine where the osteotomy will exit on the lateral side. The more proximal part of the osteotomy will exit the tibia more posteriorly and taper more anteriorly as it courses distally. The maximum obliquity possible is approximately 60° so that the osteotomy exits just anterior to the lateral intermuscular septum. This is a tapering cut from the medial border of the patellar tendon insertion to the tibial crest approximately 8 cm distally. A specially designed retractor is used to protect the lateral soft tissues as well as the neurovascular structures posterior to the lateral intermuscular septum. A power saw is used to make the initial oblique cut, and the final cuts are performed using hand osteotomes (Fig. 8, *F* and *G*). Open direct visualization of these cutting instruments as they exit laterally is imperative. A transverse cut is made just proximal to the patellar tendon with a 0.5-in straight osteotome, and a connecting cut is made between the transverse cut and the longitudinal osteotomy posterior to the tibial tubercle at its proximal extent to prevent propagation into the tibial plateau (Fig. 8, *H* and *I*).

FIGURE 7

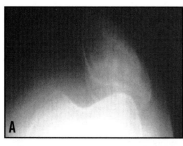
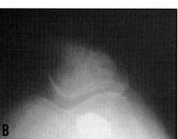

A 41-year-old woman with right patellofemoral knee pain and lateral facet arthrosis had previously undergone anterior cruciate ligament reconstruction. **A,** Preoperative 30° axial radiograph demonstrates patellar subluxation and excessive tilt. **B,** Postoperative 30° axial view demonstrates correction of patellar tilt and subluxation.

The osteotomy is carefully completed from proximal to distal using a small hand osteotome, leaving the distal soft tissues intact as much as possible. Once the osteoclasis is complete, the tubercle is rotated anteriorly and medially the desired amount (Fig. 8, *J*). The two proposed screw sites are marked on the anterior tibial cortex, and the osteotomy is fixed temporarily at the planned distal screw site with a 3.2-mm AO drill bit drilled through the osteotomy and the anterior cortex of the tibia but not through the posterior cortex. At this point the patellar tracking and correction of the Q angle are assessed clinically (Fig. 8, *K*). If the tubercle position is adequate and the patellar tracking is normal, final fixation is performed using two bicortical 4.5-mm AO cortical screws with metal washers. Leaving the distal drill bit in place, the proximal screw is inserted. The distal drill bit is then advanced carefully through the posterior cortex, and the second screw and washer are inserted (Fig. 8, *L* through *O*).

We usually perform the open part of the procedure under tourniquet control. The tourniquet is deflated prior to closure, and hemostasis is achieved carefully. We believe it is important to drain anteromedializations because the large area of exposed bone can cause significant bleeding. Furthermore, release of the tourniquet is important to ensure that no compromise of the capillary circulation to the skin occurs with closure of the wound. In general, anteriorization limited to 12 to 15 mm has not been associated with skin circulatory problems. If the patient has preexisting scars and incisions or vascular compromise, however, skin circulation should be assessed carefully. If there is any evidence of excessive pressure on the skin from the shift of the tubercle, the anteriorization should be decreased accordingly; however, this is usually not necessary. Finally, careful closure of the subcutaneous tissue and skin is performed; the fascia is never closed. A locked brace is used to immobilize the knee in a straight leg position. Overnight hospitalization is recommended; the drain is removed before discharge. After 2 to 3 days, after allowing swelling in the soft tissues to subside, a continuous passive motion machine is used at home for progressive range of motion. Early goals of physical therapy are to regain range of motion and quadriceps control.

High stress forces are placed on the tibia with an oblique osteotomy; therefore, no weight bearing is recommended for 6 weeks postoperatively. The more vertical the cut, the higher the stress risers, so that with a maximum oblique cut at 60°, no weight bearing for 6 weeks is essential. With lesser degrees of obliquity, weight bearing can most likely be allowed a little earlier. Quadriceps isometrics are encouraged early, but no resistive exercises are allowed until approximately 2 months postoperatively, to allow for osseous healing.

Results

As in most procedures, proper patient selection is critical to the success of this procedure. Several studies have documented that this procedure is very beneficial to the patient with arthrosis-associated malalignment, particularly with lateral or distal disease.[19,38,41,45,46]

ANTERIORIZATION OF THE TIBIAL TUBERCLE

There are occasional cases where medialization should be avoided in combination with anteriorization of the tibial tubercle; however, it is considered a rare case where no medialization can be tolerated. The best example is a knee that has poor lateral restraints and that has undergone a previous extensive lateral release such that medialization may cause iatrogenic medial patellar instability, which is usually a worse problem than the initial condition. This is seen in combination with a knee with no tilt or subluxation of the patella and symptomatic disease of the distal portion of the patella that has been unresponsive to nonsurgical or minor surgical procedures. It is also important that the knee have good medial restraints. Again, this occurs in a rare subset of patients. In 1994, Schepsis and associates[50] reported other indications for unloading or anteriorization of the tibial tubercle. The first patients commonly seen in the 1980s were those who had undergone a Hauser procedure in the 1970s. In the Hauser procedure, the tibial tubercle is transposed medially as well as posteriorly, and although it corrected symptoms of patellar instability, many years later patients became increasingly symptomatic from progressive patellofemoral arthrosis secondary to the increased contact pressures from moving the tibial tubercle posteriorly. In these cases, the tibial tubercle was moved back anteriorly, but because the tubercle was already medialized, further medialization could not be performed. Young, active patients who reported pain and weakness after patellectomy also had a good outcome with anteriorization. In these patients, the anteriorization improved the lever arm of the quadriceps, negating some of the negative effects of the patellectomy as well as relieving the contact pressures of the extensor mechanism on the trochlea. In many of

FIGURE 8 (A-I)

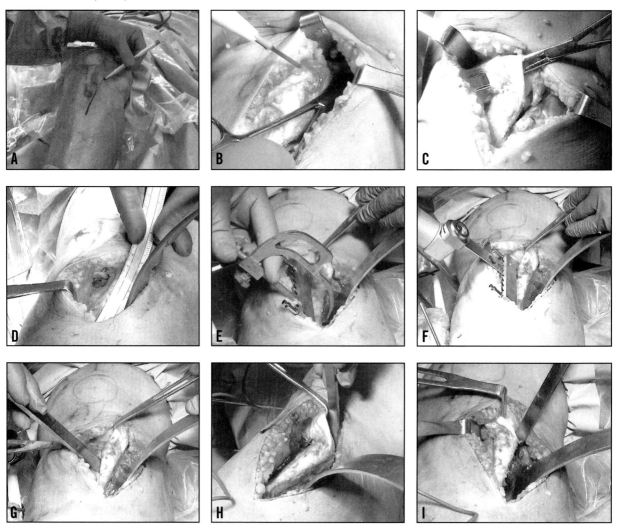

Anteromedialization procedure. **A,** Lateral incision. Care must be taken to identify previous incisions or wounds, which could impair skin circulation. **B,** A lateral release may be necessary to decrease lateral tethering. **C,** The patellar tendon is exposed and freed on both sides to allow unrestrained shift of the patella with tubercle transfer. **D,** An 8-cm-long tubercle shingle is planned. **E,** The AMZ guide (DePuy-Mitek, Norwood, MA) in position on the medial tibial slope. A caliper is used to identify the exit point of the saw blade on the lateral side. Care must be taken to ensure that the blade exits anterior to the lateral intermuscular septum. **F,** The osteotomy is initiated with an oscillating saw. A special retractor is used to protect the anterolateral musculature, which has been elevated off the lateral tibial slope subperiosteally. **G,** The initial cut is completed with an osteotome distally as it tapers toward the anterior cortex. **H,** A transverse cut is made just proximal to the insertion to the patellar tendon. **I,** An oblique cut is made to connect the transverse and longitudinal cuts and prevent propagation of the osteotomy into the tibial plateau.

these cases, "trochleamalacia" (ie, chondromalacia of the trochlea) was seen secondary to erosion of the extensor mechanism in the trochlear groove. A final group of patients who benefited from anteriorization were those with patella infera, or patella baja, where anterior or superior displacement of the tibial tubercle was necessary to bring the patella back to its normal position as well as to relieve contact pressures on the patella. Finally, tibial tubercle anteriorization can be combined with high tibial osteotomy when there is not only unicompartmental tibiofemoral disease but symptomatic patellofemoral arthrosis in a distal location.

FIGURE 8 (J-O)

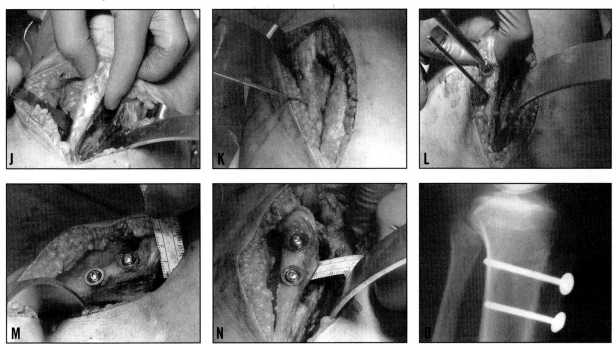

J, The tubercle shingle is now free to be shifted anteromedially along the oblique osteotomy plane. Note that the shingle remains attached distally by periosteum and soft tissue. **K,** The location of two 4.5-mm bicortical screws is marked. The tubercle is temporarily fixed distally with a 3.2-mm AO drill bit inserted to, but not through, the posterior cortex. With the tubercle fixed here, the knee is moved through its range of motion and the patellofemoral tracking is observed. **L,** If patellofemoral tracking is deemed adequate, the tubercle is fixed with the proximal and then distal screws and metal washers. These screws are placed with the knee flexed 90° to protect the posterior neurovascular structures, which are at risk with posterior cortex penetration. **M,** The amount of anteriorization is measured upon completion of the transfer. Anteriorization is generally limited to 12 to 15 mm but must be individualized based on the patient's symptoms and location of chondral lesions. **N,** Medialization is measured. Again, the amount of medialization must be individualized, depending on the amount of preoperative tubercle malalignment. **O,** Lateral radiograph of a completed anteromedialization.

FIGURE 9

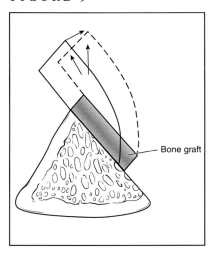

Tibial tubercle anteriorization by combining oblique osteotomy with an offset bone block. *(Reproduced with permission from Lippincott-William, and Wilkins. Fulkerson, ed 3.)*

The technique of straight anteriorization, described by Schepsis and associates,[50] uses a horizontal 10-cm-long shingle osteotomy that is kept attached distally and hinged up and supported with an autogenous bicortical iliac bone graft. Anteriorization of 12 to 15 mm was used in these cases. An alternative to this, described by Fulkerson,[1] is a maximally oblique anterior medialization cut that uses an offset bone graft to keep the anteriorization but eliminates the medialization of the tibial tubercle (Fig. 9). In general, straight anteriorization is unlikely to be successful unless very stringent and strict criteria are followed. Therefore, we use it only occasionally in our practice.

CONCLUSIONS

Tibial tubercle transfer, either in a medial, anteromedial, or anterior direction, may play a valuable role in the treatment of the patient with symptomatic patellofemoral arthrosis associated with malalignment and/or instability. Patient selection is absolutely critical to the success of these procedures, and with careful attention to technique and rehabilitation, in most cases a successful outcome will be the final result.

REFERENCES

1. Fulkerson J: *Disorders of the Patellofemoral Joint.* Baltimore, MD, William & Wilkins, 1997.

2. Merchant A, Mercer R, Jacobsen R, Cool C: Roentgenographic analysis of patellofemoral congruence. *J Bone Joint Surg Am* 1974;56:1391-1396.

3. Laurin C, Dussault R, Levesque HP: The tangential x-ray investigation of the patellofemoral joint. *Clin Orthop* 1979;144:16-26.

4. Guzzanti V, Gigante A, Di Lazzaro A, Fabbriciani C: Patellofemoral malalignment in adolescents: Computerized tomographic assessment with or without quadriceps contraction. *Am J Sports Med* 1994;22:55-60.

5. Jones R, Bartlett E, Vanright J, et al: CT determination of tibial tubercle lateralization in patients presenting with anterior knee pain. *Skeletal Radiol* 1995;24:505-509.

6. Muneta T, Yamamoto H, Ishibashi T, Asahina S, Furuya K: Computerized tomographic analysis of tibial tubercle position in the painful female patellofemoral joint. *Am J Sports Med* 1994;22:67-71.

7. Shea K, Fulkerson J: Preoperative computerized tomography scanning and arthroscopy in predicting outcome after lateral retinacular release. *Arthroscopy* 1992;8:327-334.

8. Cohen Z, Henry J, McCarthy D, Mow V, Ateshian G: Computer simulations of patellofemoral joint surgery: Patient-specific models for tuberosity transfer. *Am J Sports Med* 2003;31:87-98.

9. Dejour H, Walch G, Nove-Josserand L, Guier C: Factors of patellar instability: An anatomic radiographic study. *Knee Surg Sports Traumatol Arthrosc* 1994;2:19-26.

10. Kolowich P, Paulos L, Rosenberg T, Farnsworth S: Lateral release of the patella: Indications and contraindications. *Am J Sports Med* 1990;18:359-365.

11. Beaconsfield T, Hons B, Pintore E, et al: Radiologic measurements in patellofemoral disorders: A review. *Clin Orthop* 1994;308:18-28.

12. Benvenuti J, Rakotomanana L, Leyvraz P, Pioletti D, Heegaard J, Genton M: Displacements of the tibial tuberosity: Effects of the surgical parameters. *Clin Orthop* 1997;1:224-234.

13. Brown D, Alexander A, Lichtman D: The Elmslie-Trillat procedure: Evaluation in patellar dislocation and subluxation. *Am J Sports Med* 1984;12:104-109.

14. Cosgarea A, Schatzke M, Seth A, Litsky A: Biomechanical analysis of flat and oblique tibial tubercle osteotomy for recurrent patellar instability. *Am J Sports Med* 1999;27:507-512.

15. Cox J: Evaluation of the Roux-Elmslie-Trillat procedure for knee extensor realignment. *Am J Sports Med* 1982;10:303-310.

16. Ferguson A, Brown T, Fu F, Rutkowski: Relief of patellofemoral contact stress by anterior displacement of the tibial tubercle. *J Bone Joint Surg Am* 1979;61:159-166.

17. Ferguson A: Elevation of the insertion of the patellar ligament for patellofemoral pain. *J Bone Joint Surg Am* 1982;64:766-771.

18. Ferrandez L, Usabiaga J, Yubero J, Sagarra J, de No L: An experimental study of the redistribution of patellofemoral pressures by anterior displacement of the anterior tuberosity of the tibia. *Clin Orthop* 1989;283:183-189.

19. Fulkerson J, Becker G, Meaney J, Miranda M, Folcik M: Anteromedial tibial tubercle transfer without bone graft. *Am J Sports Med* 1990;18:490-496.

20. Hungerford D, Barry M: Biomechanics of the patellofemoral joint. *Clin Orthop* 1979;144:9-15.

21. Nakamura T: Advancement of tibial tuberosity: A biomechanical study. *J Bone Joint Surg Br* 1985;67:255.

22. Naranja R, Reilly P, Kuhlman J, Haut E, Torg J: Long-term evaluation of the Elmslie-Trillat-Maquet procedure for patellofemoral dysfunction. *Am J Sports Med* 1996;24:779-784.

23. Pan HQ, Kish V, Boyd RD, Burr DB, Radin EL: The Maquet procedure: Effect of tibial shingle length on patellofemoral pressures. *J Orthop Res* 1993;11:199-204.

24. Radin E: The Maquet procedure-anterior displacement of the tibial tubercle: Indications, contraindications, and precautions. *Clin Orthop* 1986;213:241.

25. Radin E: Anterior tibial tubercle elevation in the young adult. *Orthop Clin North Am* 1986;17:297.

26. Radin E, Pan H: Long-term follow-up study on the Maquet procedure with special references to the causes of failure. *Clin Orthop* 1993;290:253-258.

27. Shelbourne K, Porter D, Rozzi W: Use of a modified Elmslie-Trillat procedure to improve abnormal patellar congruence angle. *Am J Sports Med* 1994;22:318-323.

28. Kuroda R, Kambic H, Valdevit A, Andrish J: Articular cartilage contact pressures after tibial tubercle transfer. *Am J Sports Med* 2001;29:403-409.

29. Trillat A, Dejour H, Couette A: Diagnostic et traitement des subluxation recidivantes de la rotule. *Rev Chir Orthop* 1964;50:813.

30. Farr J: Distal realignment for recurrent patellar instability: Operative techniques in patellar instability. *Sports Med* 2001;9:176-182.

31. Maquet P: A biomechanical treatment of femoro-patellar arthrosis: Advancement of the patellar tendon. *Rev Rhum Mal Osteoartic* 1963;30:779-783.

32. Maquet P: Advancement of the tibial tuberosity. *Clin Orthop* 1976;115:225.

33. Maquet P: Mechanics and osteoarthritis of the patellofemoral joint. *Clin Orthop* 1979;144:70-73.

34. Maquet P: *Biomechanics of the Knee,* ed 2. Berlin, Germany, Springer-Verlag, 1984.

35. Bandi W: Chondromalacia patella und femo-patellare arthrose. *Helv Chir Acta* 1972;1:3.

36. Bellemans J, Cauwenberghs F, Witvrouw E, Brys P, Victor J: Anteromedial tibial tubercle transfer in patients with chronic anterior knee pain and a subluxation type patella malalignment. *Am J Sports Med* 1997;25:375-381.

37. Bessette G, Hunter R: The Maquet procedure: A retrospective view. *Clin Orthop* 1998;232:159-167.

38. Fulkerson J: Anteromedialization of the tibial tuberosity for patellofemoral malalignment. *Clin Orthop* 1983;177: 176-181.

39. Heatley FW, Allen PR, Patrick JH: Tibial tubercle advancement for anterior knee pain. *Clin Orthop* 1986;208:215-224.

40. Hirsch D: Experience with Maquet anterior tibial tubercle advancement for patellofemoral arthralgia. *Clin Orthop* 1980;148:136.

41. Koshino T: Changes in patellofemoral compressive force after anterior or anteromedial displacement of tibial tuberosity for chondromalacia patella. *Clin Orthop* 1991; 266:133.

42. Leach R, Radin E: Anterior displacement of the tibial tubercle for patellofemoral arthrosis. *Orthop Trans* 1979; 3:291.

43. Leach R, Schepsis A: Anterior displacement of the tibial tubercle: The Maquet procedure. *Contemporary Orthop* 1981;3:199.

44. Lund F, Nilsson BE: Anterior displacement of tibial tuberosity in chondromalacia patella. Acta *Orthop Scand* 1980;51:679-688.

45. Pidoriano A, Weinstein R, Buuck D, Fulkerson J: Correlation of patellar articular lesions with results from anteromedial tibial tubercle transfer. *Am J Sports Med* 1997;25: 533-537.

46. Post W, Fulkerson J: Distal realignment of the patellofemoral joint. *Orthop Clin North Am* 1992;23: 631-643.

47. Putnam M, Mears D, Fu F: Combined Maquet and proximal tibial valgus osteotomy. *Clin Orthop* 1985;197:217-223.

48. Rappaport L, et al: The Maquet osteotomy. *Orthop Clin North Am* 1992;23:634-656.

49. Rozbruch J, et al: Tibial tubercle elevation: A clinical study of 31 cases. *Orthop Trans* 1979;3:291.

50. Schepsis A, et al: Anterior tibial tubercle transposition for patellofemoral arthrosis: A long-term study. *Am J Knee Surg* 1994;l:7.

51. Schmid F: The Maquet procedure in the treatment of patellofemoral osteoarthritis. *Clin Orthop* 1993;294: 254-258.

52. Siegel M: The Maquet osteotomy: A review of risks. *Orthopedics* 1987;10:1073-1078.

53. Sudmann E, Salkowitsch B: Anterior displacement of tibial tuberosity in the treatment of chondromalacia patella. *Acta Orthop Scand* 1980;51:679.

54. Waisbrod H, Treiman N: Anterior displacement of tibial tuberosity for patellofemoral disorders. *Clin Orthop* 1980; 153:180-182.

ISOLATED PATELLOFEMORAL ARTHRITIS WITHOUT MALALIGNMENT

GWO-CHIN LEE, MD

MICHAEL A. KELLY, MD

Knee pain secondary to degeneration of the patellofemoral joint is a common musculoskeletal problem. When associated with tibiofemoral arthritis, total knee arthroplasty has been shown effective in improving pain and function.[1,2] Treatment of isolated patellofemoral arthritis, however, can be a challenge because the patients are often young and many have severe pain.[3,4] Although activity modifications, nonsteroidal anti-inflammatory drugs, and physical therapy play a primary role in treatment, a subset of these patients will continue to have disabling symptoms and will require surgical intervention.

Surgical treatment of patients with isolated patellofemoral arthritis largely depends on the age of the patient, the extent of patellar and trochlear involvement, and the presence of patellar instability and maltracking.[5] This chapter focuses on patients with isolated patellofemoral arthritis without patellar instability, reviews pertinent surgical techniques, and provides a logical treatment algorithm.

PATIENT EVALUATION

Treatment of the patient with anterior knee pain and radiographic evidence of isolated patellofemoral arthritis begins in the office.[6] Obtaining a complete history and physical examination is essential to precisely define the underlying pathology and provide appropriate treatment. Any history of fracture, dislocation, and surgery should be elicited. The location, quality, and onset and duration of knee pain offer important clues about its etiology. Although patients with patellofemoral disease often have anterior knee pain, patients with advanced involvement of the trochlear groove often have symptoms referred to the posterior aspect of the knee.[7]

Examination should then focus on the knee and the patella, recording any signs of crepitus, tilt, and patellar maltracking, limited knee motion, and angular deformity. Other causes of knee pain such as patellar tendinitis, prepatellar bursitis, symptomatic plica, and quadriceps tendinitis should be considered and excluded. Tenderness to palpation of the medial and lateral joint line may reveal underlying tibiofemoral degeneration or meniscal pathology. Patellar tilt should be carefully evaluated to assess patellofemoral alignment. Referred pain from the lumbosacral spine and ipsilateral hip should be ruled out.

FIGURE 1

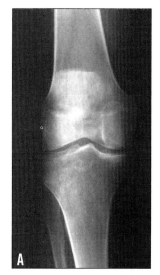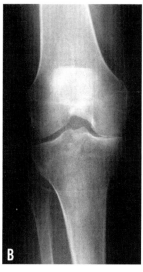

Radiographs of a knee with early osteoarthritis of the tibiofemoral joint. **A,** Weight-bearing AP view. **B,** PA flexion view with the knee in 45° of flexion shows severe narrowing of the medial compartment not seen on the AP view.

Finally, findings of patellar hypermobility and a J-sign should raise suspicions for patellar instability, which would alter the management of the patient.[8]

Radiographs are often necessary to establish a proper diagnosis and formulate an effective treatment plan. Weight-bearing AP, lateral, and modified Merchant views should be obtained. A PA radiograph with the knee in 45° of flexion is helpful in the detection of early arthritis of the tibiofemoral joint (Fig. 1). Patellofemoral arthritis normally involves the lateral facet, and an axial view will reveal narrowing of the lateral joint space of the patellofemoral articulation with evidence of osteophyte formation on the lateral patella and the trochlea (Fig. 2). Patellofemoral joint space narrowing may also be evident on the lateral view. Malalignment of the patella is best seen on axial views. CT scans obtained at varying degrees of knee flexion may sometimes reveal subtle patellar malalignment in a minority of patients with normal radiographs[9] (Fig. 3). Bone scans are also useful, especially when coexisting complex regional pain syndrome in the extremity is suspected.

NONSURGICAL TREATMENT

Patients with isolated patellofemoral arthritis present therapeutic challenges to the surgeon. They often have incapacitating knee pain that severely restricts their activities of daily living. Radiographic findings routinely appear benign and do not correlate with the severity of symptoms.[10] For younger patients with minimal radiographic evidence of arthritis, the cornerstone of successful nonsurgical treatment is improved patient understanding of the underlying problem.

Management consists of a comprehensive nonsurgical knee program that focuses on quadriceps muscle strengthening and activity modifications.[11] Use of a stationary bicycle is preferred, and impact activities such as jogging or the use of treadmills should be avoided. Most importantly, patients need to be educated. It is important to discuss the basic biomechanics of the patellofemoral joint and emphasize the importance of optimizing body weight and avoiding activities that increase forces across the patellofemoral joint such as stair climbing or squatting. Through activity modifications and improved understanding of the problem and treatment rationale, many patients with early evidence of isolated patellofemoral arthritis return to activities with minimal knee discomfort for an extended period of time.

SURGICAL TREATMENT

When nonsurgical treatment fails and the patient continues to have significant pain and disability, surgical intervention is warranted. Four categories of surgical procedures have been described for the treatment of patellofemoral arthritis: (1) arthroscopic débridement and chondroplasty with or without lateral release; (2) tibial tubercle elevation/osteotomy; (3) patellar resurfacing, patellofemoral arthroplasty, and total knee arthroplasty; and (4) patellectomy. The procedure selected depends largely on the patient's age, the extent of patellofemoral joint involvement, and other abnormalities in the knee.

FIGURE 2

FIGURE 3

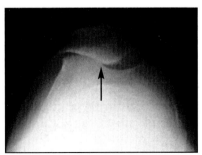

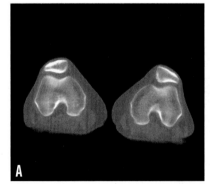
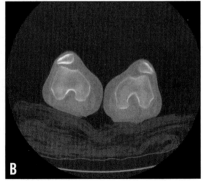

Axial view of a knee with patellofemoral arthritis. The lateral joint space of the patellofemoral articulation is narrowed, and there is evidence of osteophyte formation.

Subtle patellar instability is sometimes demonstrated with CT scans obtained at varying degrees of knee flexion. **A,** CT scan taken with the knee at 45° of flexion shows the patella centered on the trochlea. **B,** CT scan taken with the knee at 15° of knee flexion shows lateral tilt and subluxation of the patella.

Surgery
Meniscus Lesion

Arthroscopy

The role of therapeutic arthroscopy in the management of patients with patellofemoral arthritis continues to be a topic for debate. Diagnostic arthroscopy, however, is an invaluable tool in quantifying the extent of patellofemoral joint involvement and helps rule out other sources of knee pathology.

The most common arthroscopic procedure performed is a débridement with patellar shaving. The goals of this treatment are to remove any mechanical element to the patient's pain and to decrease cartilage breakdown products associated with synovitis of the knee.[12,13]

Technique

Our technique of débridement begins with conducting a standard diagnostic arthroscopic examination through standard anterior lateral and medial portals. The patellofemoral compartment is carefully assessed, and the size and extent of cartilage abnormalities involving the patella and the trochlea are documented. Superolateral portals may be used to evaluate patellofemoral tracking or to perform chondroplasty. Cartilage lesions are graded according to size, depth, and location. A conservative approach is used with respect to chondral shaving. Loose flaps and fibrillations are débrided using a motorized shaver. No attempt is made to stimulate cartilage repair with arthrosis, and care is taken not to violate the subchondral bone. The joint is then thoroughly irrigated and a compression dressing is applied. The patient resumes rehabilitation in the form of riding a stationary bike the day after surgery.

Results

Few studies have looked at the effect of limited arthroscopic débridement in patients with arthritis of the patellofemoral joint. Ogilvie-Harris and Jackson[14] reported on a group of 42 patients with posttraumatic patellofemoral changes treated with débridement and lavage. At a mean follow-up of 5 years, only 20% of patients with exposed subchondral bone had satisfactory results. More recently, Federico and Reider[15] evaluated 36 patients who underwent patellar débridement for patellofemoral pain. No patients had clinical or radiographic evidence of malalignment or instability, and all had grade 2 or worse chondromalacia at the time of surgery. At final follow-up, all but four patients reported subjective improvements in pain and function; however, only 50% of patients had good or excellent results following surgery. Other studies

have al
rates o
up.[16,17]

The
have be
propos
fibrous
and ass
posttra
arthros
tory res
howeve
and at a
tory results in only 50% of the patients. Other authors have reported that limited grade 2 and 3 changes in the knee and patient age younger than 30 years are good prognostic factors.[21,22]

Débridement of the patellofemoral articulation should be performed with care, and violation of the subchondral plate should be avoided. Biomechanical studies have shown that early cartilage lesions continue to transfer load, whereas grade 3 and 4 cartilage lesions do not.[23] Furthermore, cystic degeneration of the patella following chondroplasty and subchondral bone perforation has been reported.[24] Consequently, it is prudent to not convert partial-thickness cartilage lesions into full-thickness cartilage lesions and to be conservative in the removal of cartilage flaps unless they are unstable. The drilling of small full-thickness cartilage lesions with preservation of the surrounding cartilage rim is advocated. In larger lesions, these techniques are combined with other unloading procedures.

Lateral Release

Many surgeons believe that there is a role for lateral release in the treatment of early isolated patellofemoral arthritis. The rationale is that by releasing the lateral retinaculum, the lateral facet of the patella is unloaded from the trochlea.[25,26] Both open and arthroscopic techniques for lateral release have been well described.[27] The ideal patient has signs of early patellofemoral arthritis, tilt, and narrowing of the lateral aspect of the patellofemoral joint. Typically, these patients have localized crepitation, tenderness over the lateral patellar facet, and a tight lateral retinaculum with lateral patellar tilt. A lateral release should not be performed in patients with patellar hypermobility because of the risk of iatrogenically induced medial patellar instability.[28,29]

Lateral release in patients with patellofemoral arthritis has usually been combined with arthroscopic débridement. The reported results of this procedure have been variable. Aderinto and Cobb[30] evaluated 50 patients who underwent lateral release for treatment of patellofemoral arthritis. At a mean follow-up of 31 months, 80% of patients reported improvements in pain compared with before surgery; however, 41% of these patients were dissatisfied with their knee at last follow-up. Similarly, Jackson and associates[25] in a follow-up at 4 years, reported good or excellent results in 75% of patients with unremitting anterior knee pain who were treated with arthroscopy and lateral release; however, at 6-year follow-up, satisfactory results had deteriorated to 56%. Others studies have found severe articular damage and patient age older than 30 years to be poor prognostic factors.[31-33]

Surgical results with lateral release are unpredictable; therefore, preoperative patient counseling is crucial. Patients should be informed that while the goal of this procedure is to temporize and relieve symptoms, it does not halt disease progression. Patients with tilt and early degenerative disease are good candidates for lateral retinacular release and débridement with a good chance of success. Postoperative rehabilitation is crucial.

Tibial Tubercle Elevation/Osteotomy

Tibial tubercle elevation was originally advocated by Maquet[34] as an alternative to patellectomy in patients who failed to respond to treatment of anterior knee pain. The rationale for this procedure was to decrease the resultant force on the patellofemoral articulation by increasing the lever arm of the patellar tendon. In his original description of the procedure, Maquet calculated a 50% reduction in patellofemoral forces with a 2-cm advancement of the tibial tubercle.[35] Others have described similar procedures for unloading the patellofemoral joint.[36] In the US, Fulkerson[37] described a combination of tubercle elevation and medialization to address arthrosis and malalignment.

Basic science studies have looked at the effects of tibial tubercle elevation on patellofemoral contact forces. Ferguson and associates[38] reported that most of the reduction of forces across the patellofemoral joint occurred in the first 1.25 cm of elevation. They also noted a shift of forces to the superior pole of the patella with increasing elevation of the distal pole. Other studies have confirmed this load transfer to the proximal pole and concluded that a tubercle elevation of 1 cm is biomechanically optimal.[39,40] Finally, Fulkerson and associates[41] evaluated the

effects of anteriomedialization of the tibial tubercle in cadaver knees and reported that the load on the lateral facets decreased only in the first 0° to 30° of motion. At knee flexion greater than 30°, there was no significant reduction in forces compared with preoperative values.

A good understanding of the mechanics of this procedure and sound patient selection are essential to a successful clinical outcome. Patients with small focal distal lesions with minimal trochlear involvement may be good candidates for this procedure.[42] Patients with extensive lateral and proximal involvement of the patella may not be suitable candidates. In this circumstance, arthroplasty or patellectomy may be the only choices available to the surgeon.

Maquet Tibial Tubercle Elevation

In Maquet's original description of this procedure, the tibial tubercle is osteotomized and the osteotomy is extended approximately 12 cm distally. No internal fixation is used, and he advocates anterior displacement of the tibial tubercle by at least 2 cm using a wedged block of iliac crest bone graft.[43]

Using a long anterolateral skin incision extending from the superior pole of the patella to the distal aspect of the proposed osteotomy, an open lateral retinacular release is performed and the lateral geniculate vessels are ligated. The anterior compartment of the calf is exposed and released. The exposure allows good visualization of the patellar tendon insertion and the tibial crest, and care must be taken to develop full-thickness skin flaps during exposure. The osteotomy is performed at a depth of approximately 8 mm posterior to the tibial crest using either an osteotome or an oscillating saw. Two osteotomes inserted at the medial and lateral aspects of the osteotomy are driven in an alternate fashion and the tibial tubercle is gradually elevated. The distal periosteal hinge must be preserved during elevation of the tibial tubercle. Overall, the length of the osteotomy is approximately 10 cm. Using a bone block harvested from the iliac crest, the tibial tubercle is then elevated approximately 10 to 15 mm (Fig. 4). The graft is placed at the tip of the tibial tubercle. More distal graft placement has been associated with fractures of the proximal aspect of the tibial tubercle. The remaining area posterior to the osteotomy is filled in with morcellized bone graft.

The bone graft is typically stable without internal fixation. Fracture of the distal cortex of the osteotomy may necessitate the use of screw fixation. The fascia is not closed. The wound is closed, taking great care to avoid

FIGURE 4

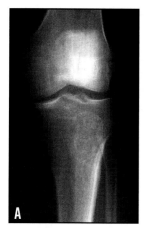 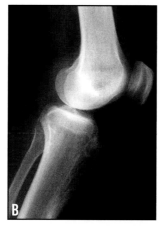

Radiographs of the knee of a patient 10 years after a Maquet tibial tubercle elevation. AP **(A)** and lateral **(B)** views.

excessive skin tension with closure. Proper wound healing is critical to the success of this procedure and takes priority in the early postoperative recovery period. The knee is splinted in extension until the wound heals, at which time partial weight bearing and gentle motion are permitted. Aggressive rehabilitation based on closed-chain exercises is started at 6 weeks postoperatively.

Results of the Maquet Procedure

Maquet[44] reported on 37 knees treated with isolated tibial tubercle elevation, at an average follow-up of 4.7 years. At last follow-up, 36 knees had satisfactory results. One knee had skin necrosis requiring removal of the bone graft. Jenny and associates[45] evaluated 100 patients with chondromalacia patella treated with a Maquet tibial tubercle elevation. At 4-year follow-up, the overall satisfaction rate was 62%. Reevaluation of 65 of the original 100 patients at 11 years showed that the overall success rate remained unchanged at 62%. No specific mention was made about the outcome of patients lost to follow-up. Radin and Pan[46] reported similar results in a group of 42 patients with symptomatic osteoarthritis of the patellofemoral joint. At an average 6-year follow-up, 79% had a satisfactory outcome, the major complication rate was 7%, and other failures were attributed to unrecognized arthritis of the tibiofemoral joint and social or psychiatric reasons.

Significant morbidity is associated with this procedure, and various authors have reported a variety of complications, the most common following surgery being skin complications. Mendes and associates[47] reported sig-

FIGURE 5

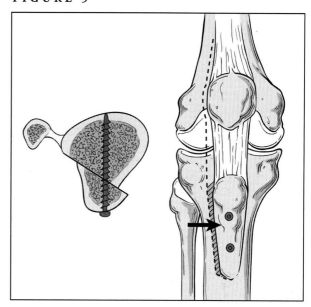

Fulkerson anteromedial tubercle transfer. The obliquity of the osteotomy plane can be varied to alter the relative amount of medial and anterior displacement of the tibial tubercle. As the obliquity of the osteotomy increases, more anterior displacement can be obtained.

nificant wound complications in 8 of 25 patients and an overall complication rate of 55%. Ferguson[48] reported that limiting the amount of elevation resulted in decreased wound complications. Bessette and Hunter[49] and Putz and associates[50] reported graft problems, nonunions, and tibial fractures as a result of this procedure.

Fulkerson Anteromedial Tubercle Transfer

Fulkerson[51] originally described an anteromedial tibial tubercle transfer as a procedure to address both patellar arthritis and malalignment. Unlike Maquet's procedure for tibial tubercle elevation, Fulkerson described an oblique osteotomy that accomplishes elevation and medial transfer without the need for bone graft. By changing the angle of obliquity, the surgeon can choose to emphasize either medialization (to address instability) or anterior elevation (to unload the patellofemoral joint) as deemed appropriate (Fig. 5).

The Fulkerson anteromedialization consists of a midline incision and an open lateral release. The proximal portion of the anterior compartment of the leg is exposed and the tibialis anterior origin is elevated with electrocautery. The patellar tendon insertion is protected. An oblique osteotomy is done from anteromedial to posterolateral and tapered over 6 to 7 cm from the proximal insertion of the patellar tendon, using care to preserve a distal osteoperiosteal hinge. In patients without significant malalignment, a specific steep osteotomy is used to anteriorize the tubercle. The proposed angle of the osteotomy is marked with drill bits or Steinmann pins and the osteotomy is completed with a saw. Some surgeons prefer to make multiple perforations with a drill and complete the work with an osteotome. A vertical cut is made just proximal to the patellar tendon insertion to free the tubercle fragment that is then moved medially and anteriorly up the inclined plane formed by the oblique osteotomy. Excellent fixation can be obtained with two 4.5-mm cortical screws that are countersunk and placed bicortically.

Provided that good fixation has been obtained, patients are encouraged to pursue active assisted and passive range of motion of 90° to 100° in the first 6 weeks after surgery. The leg is protected in a hinged knee brace, and patients are allowed to ambulate with partial weight bearing for the first 6 weeks. At 6 weeks, a quadriceps strengthening program that emphasizes closed-chain kinetic exercises is started.[52] Weight bearing is increased when satisfactory healing of the osteotomy is evident; the precise timing is variable.

Results of the Fulkerson Procedure

The results of the Fulkerson technique are similar to those reported for the Maquet procedure but with lower complication rates, particularly wound problems. Fulkerson and associates[41] reported a patient satisfaction rate of 93% in 30 patients at 2-year follow-up. Subsequent reexamination of a limited number of patients at 5 years found that all maintained the good result. In patients with severe patellofemoral arthritis, however, only 75% had good results and none had excellent results. There were no reported complications of skin necrosis, compartment syndrome, or infection. Morshuis and associates[53] reported similar results in a series of 25 knees treated with anteromedialization of the tubercle. At 12-month follow-up, 84% had satisfactory results, but at 38 months, the satisfactory results had deteriorated to 70%. The best results were obtained in knees with patellofemoral pain and no signs of medial proximal patellofemoral arthritis. No skin or tubercle complications were reported in this series.

There are several advantages to the Fulkerson procedure. Bone grafting is not required; therefore, the mor-

bidity associated with autogenous bone graft harvest is eliminated. More importantly, the reported rates of skin complications are lower than those reported for other unloading procedures. The most common complications following the Fulkerson procedure are joint hemiarthrosis from the lateral release and hematoma bleeding from the osteotomy site.[54] Other risks inherent in the Fulkerson technique are damage to the anterior tibial artery and deep peroneal nerve. Less common complications include loss of fixation, delayed union or nonunion,[55] tibial shaft fracture,[56] patella baja, and pain from prominent hardware. A tibial fracture at the distal aspect of a healed tibial osteotomy with minor trauma was reported at 5 months following surgery. The initial concerns regarding stiffness following this procedure have been largely eliminated with the use of early continuous passive motion and range-of-motion exercises.

Both the Maquet and Fulkerson procedures are technically demanding and are associated with significant morbidity; therefore, careful patient selection is crucial to a successful clinical outcome. Young patients with focal distal patellar lesions and mild trochlear changes may be considered candidates for this procedure. Older patients with diffuse patellar and trochlear involvement may be

FIGURE 6

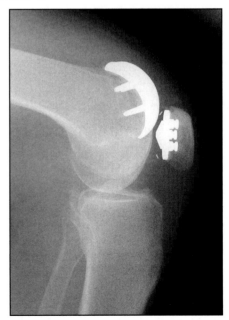

Lateral radiograph of a patellofemoral arthroplasty.

better served by more conservative treatment options that will not compromise the results of future total knee arthroplasty.

Patellar Hemiarthroplasty and Patellofemoral Arthroplasty

Patellar hemiarthroplasty and patellofemoral arthroplasty (Fig. 6) can be considered in the younger patient with severe arthritis and can serve as alternatives to patellectomy. In older patients with severe isolated patellofemoral arthritis, total knee arthroplasty is effective at relieving pain and improving function. Surgical decision making, however, is much more difficult in younger patients with advanced patellofemoral degenerative changes. As previously mentioned, patients with involvement of the proximal pole of the patella and severe arthritis of the trochlea are not good candidates for tibial tubercle elevation. Although several studies have shown that total knee arthroplasty is durable in young patients, there are valid reservations within the orthopaedic community about performing total knee arthroplasties in patients younger than 50 years.[57-59] Recently, there has been renewed interest in patellar hemiarthroplasty and patellofemoral arthroplasty. The proposed advantages are bone conservation and an easy conversion to subsequent total knee arthroplasty. Although these procedures both are performed sparingly in the US, several designs and implant options are available. Patellofemoral arthroplasty is performed more routinely in Europe.

Technique

The surgical technique for patellar hemiarthroplasty is similar to that used in a standard total knee arthroplasty. Obtaining proper balance and alignment of the extensor mechanism is critical. The goal is to restore near-normal patellar mechanics following implantation of the patellar prosthesis. Although the optimal prosthesis design is debatable, attention to the thickness of the patella at resurfacing appears to be important because overstuffing of the patellofemoral joint has been shown to have a deleterious effect on patellar tracking.[60,61] My colleagues and I recommend making the composite thickness no greater than the original patellar thickness. This procedure would seem to have rare indications when the articular degeneration is limited to the patella, such as in a posttraumatic condition.

Patellofemoral arthroplasty is performed through an anterior midline incision and medial parapatellar arthro-

tomy. The trochlea is inspected, and notch osteophytes are removed to prevent impingement on the tibial spines. Depending on the type of implant, the trochlea is fashioned either manually or with the aid of instrumentation to accept the trochlear implant. Recent modifications have improved the instrumentation techniques and have improved the ease of patellofemoral resurfacing. Care must be taken not to tilt the prosthesis. The tip of the trochlear component should not overhang into the notch because this will cause impingement against the tibial spines. The patellar component is then implanted, with care taken to restore the normal patellar thickness. Extensor mechanism realignment is necessary to ensure proper patellar tracking. This is a critical part of the procedure. The knee should be put through a range of motion. If there is catching past 110° or if patella baja is noted, some authors recommend a concurrent proximal transfer of the tibial tubercle.[62] Impingement proximally in early flexion and notch impingement with increasing knee flexion must be avoided.

Results

Overall, the results of patellar hemiarthroplasty have been unpredictable. Since McKeever,[63] Depalma and associates,[64] and Levitt[65] reported on their initial results, patient satisfaction following this procedure has ranged from 50% to 80%. Insall and associates[66] reported on 29 patients who were implanted with a second-generation patellar prosthesis developed at the Hospital for Special Surgery. At 3- to 6-year follow-up, only 55% of the patients had good or excellent results. Satisfactory results were reported in 67% with no tibiofemoral arthritis. Other authors have linked inferior results with degenerative changes at the femoral and tibial surfaces noted at the time of surgery.[67]

Recently there has been renewed interest in using patellofemoral arthroplasty to treat patients with severe arthritis isolated to the patellofemoral joint. Although most modern experience has been outside the US, there have been a few studies on the long-term results of patellofemoral arthroplasty. Kooijman and associates[68] reported on the outcome of 45 Richards patellofemoral arthroplasties at a mean follow-up of 17 years. The authors found that 86% of patients had good to excellent results, with a loosening rate of 2%, and 10 patients underwent subsequent conversion to total knee arthroplasty at a mean of 15 years with minimal difficulty. Inferior results with higher complication rates have been reported with other implant designs. Tauro and associates[69] reported on 59 patients (76 knees) treated with arthroplasty using the first-generation Lubinus prosthesis and found a 28% revision rate (21 knees) and a satisfactory outcome in only 45% of patients at a mean follow-up of 7.5 years. Maltracking of the patella, resulting in tilt and polyethelyne wear, was the most common complication in this group. The Avon group has since redesigned its prosthesis, and a recent report by Ackroyd and associates[70] reported significant improvements in patient satisfaction and significantly lower loosening and complication rates.

In our practice, the role of patellar hemiarthroplasty is very limited. In patients who are candidates for arthroplasty of the patellofemoral compartment, we recommend both trochlear and patellar resurfacing. Newer implant designs for patellofemoral arthroplasty hold promise in providing successful long-term pain relief with lower complication rates.

Total Knee Arthroplasty

Surgical treatment of isolated patellofemoral arthritis remains controversial and presents a challenging treatment dilemma. Patellectomy,[71] lateral retinacular release, and cartilage implantation have had limited success in the treatment of this condition.[72] The results of isolated patellofemoral arthroplasty have been variable. In older patients, total knee arthroplasty is a viable option, particularly when there are degenerative changes in other compartments.

Laskin and van Stejin[73] reported on the short-term outcome of 53 patients with isolated patellofemoral arthritis who were treated with total knee arthroplasty and compared the results with a concomitant series of patients with tricompartmental osteoarthritis. The procedure predictably provided excellent pain relief and improvement in function; however, a higher percentage of patients had evidence of postoperative patellar tilt, and there was a threefold increase in the need for lateral retinacular release at the time of total knee arthroplasty. Similarly, Parvizi and associates[74] evaluated 31 total knee arthroplasties performed in 24 patients with advanced patellofemoral arthritis. At a mean follow-up of 5.2 years, there was significant improvement in pain and function. Twenty-one knees required a lateral retinacular release, and three knees required additional formal proximal realignment at the time of total knee arthroplasty.

These results emphasize the challenges of optimizing patellar tracking in total knee arthroplasty. Despite improvements in surgical technique and prosthetic design, patellofemoral complications following total knee arthroplasty remain a leading cause of revision.[75-77] Total knee arthroplasty in patients with severe patellofemoral arthritis poses particular challenges to the orthopaedic surgeon. The lateral facet of the patella is often worn asymmetrically; therefore, even resurfacing of the patella is crucial. In addition, femoral and tibial component rotation must be correct to optimize patellofemoral tracking. We attempt to position the femoral component parallel to the transepicondylar axis of the femur at the time of arthroplasty.[78,79] The intercondylar femoral line is a good secondary rotational landmark.[80] The tibial component should be positioned at the junction of the middle and medial third of the tibial tubercle. Excessive internal rotation of the tibial component effectively increases the Q angle and can lead to patellar instability following total knee arthroplasty. Lateral release and proximal realignment may be necessary to rebalance the extensor mechanism. Finally, "overstuffing" of the patellofemoral joint must be avoided. We recommend that the patella-prosthesis composite not exceed the thickness of the native patella.[81] All these steps must be taken to ensure a successful outcome following total knee arthroplasty (Fig. 7).

Patellectomy

Patellectomy has long been used in the management of intractable patellofemoral pain. It is typically considered a salvage procedure for young patients with advanced degenerative disease of the patella. Various surgical techniques for patellectomy have been well described in the orthopaedic literature.[82,83] Reconstruction of the remaining extensor mechanism is essential to a successful out-

FIGURE 7

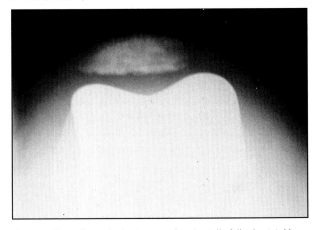

Postoperative radiograph showing resurfaced patella following total knee arthroplasty. A well-centered and symmetrically resurfaced patellar component is the key to a successful clinical outcome.

come. Gunal and associates[84] proposed closing the defect longitudinally and advancing a strip of the vastus medialis obliquus distally and laterally by 1 cm. The authors noted that this technique led to improved cosmesis and range of motion and only mild loss of power when compared with results in patients treated with simple patellectomy. Furthermore, care must be taken to balance the residual extensor mechanism and ensure its proper engagement in the trochlea in knee flexion. Occasionally, formal realignment of the extensor mechanism needs to be performed. We prefer the surgical technique for patellectomy described by Compere and associates.[85] Through an anterior midline incision, the patella is carefully enucleated to preserve the extensor mechanism. The remaining extensor mechanism is tabularized and proper tracking of the "tube" is ensured. Proper strengthening is a lengthy process following this procedure; therefore, early range of motion should be initiated. In our limited experience, this technique has been preferred by patients for cosmesis and function.

The importance of the patella in normal knee biomechanics is well documented, but conflicting reports exist in the literature regarding the clinical outcome following patellectomy.[86,87] Kelly and Insall[88] reviewed 100 patellectomies used to treat arthritis or patellar fractures and found good to excellent results in 72%. Failure was almost always the result of unrelieved pain and associated with tibiofemoral disease. Lennox and associates[89] reported on the knee function of 69 patients following 83 patellectomies with a minimum follow-up of 12 years. In their series, only 54% of patients who were treated for patellofemoral arthritis achieved good clinical results, and the average quadriceps strength was 60% of the contralateral side. The main source of failure was attributed to progression of disease in the other compartments of the knee. Other studies have shown degenerative changes in the other trochlea and tibiofemoral articulation as leading causes of failure following patellectomy. Feller and Bartlett[90] reported that 15 of 16 patients with poor outcomes following patellectomy had significant articular degeneration of the medial compartment and the trochlear groove.

Based on these findings, a careful and complete evaluation of the entire knee must be performed prior to patellectomy. The goal is to try to save the patella when possible and look for other treatment options. In our opinion, patellectomy has a limited role and may be indicated in very young patients with severe patellar arthritis. Signifi-

cant arthrosis of the trochlea and other compartments of the knee is a contraindication for this procedure. Furthermore, alterations in knee biomechanics that occur following surgery may compromise the results of subsequent total knee arthroplasty.

CONCLUSIONS

Isolated patellofemoral arthritis continues to be a difficult problem to treat. The treatment needs to be individually tailored to the patient and depends largely on the age of the patient, extent of patellofemoral joint involvement, and other abnormalities. In patients with minimal disease, a comprehensive nonsurgical treatment program that focuses on activity modifications is usually successful in returning patients to near-normal function. For patients whose symptoms do not respond to nonsurgical treatment, arthroscopy can be a useful initial step in defining the extent of patellofemoral joint involvement and ruling out other causes of joint derangement. Débridement should be conservative, and the surgeon should avoid converting partial-thickness lesions to full-thickness lesions. Patients with early arthritis and radiographic evidence of patellar tilt may benefit from a concurrent lateral release.

Young patients with focal distal lesions and minimal trochlear involvement may benefit from tibial tubercle elevation. This procedure alters patellofemoral contact forces and is designed to unload the patella from the trochlea; however, it is associated with significant morbidity and the postoperative recovery period is substantial. In patients who are candidates for tubercle elevation, we prefer an anteromedialization procedure as described by Fulkerson,[37] performing a steep osteotomy to primarily anteriorize the tubercle. These patients should be counseled and educated preoperatively so that their expectations are realistic. The procedure should not be performed in older patients because it may compromise future results of knee arthroplasty.

Recently, there has been renewed interest in isolated patellofemoral joint arthroplasty. This procedure attempts to address the pathology and to minimize bone resection. Although early results of newer designs of patellofemoral prostheses show significant reductions in pain and lower complication rates, wide adoption of this technique as a treatment for severe isolated patellofemoral arthritis is still far away. In select patients, patellofemoral arthroplasty can provide significant pain relief and bridge the temporal gap until knee arthroplasty is needed.

In patients older than 50 years, we believe that total knee arthroplasty should be performed when the patient has exhausted more conservative therapeutic options. To date, knee arthroplasty continues to be reliable, durable, and effective in improving pain and function in patients with degenerative joint disease. Several studies have demonstrated the effectiveness of this procedure. Optimizing patellofemoral tracking can be a challenge in these patients. The surgeon must be aware of all the pitfalls and pay close attention to details to obtain a total knee arthroplasty with a balanced extensor mechanism.

References

1. Vince KG, McPherson EJ: The patella in total knee arthroplasty. *Orthop Clin North Am* 1992;23:675-686.
2. Insall JN, Tria AJ, Aglietti P: Resurfacing of the patella. *J Bone Joint Surg Am* 1980;62:933-936.
3. McAlindon TE, Snow S, Cooper C, et al: Radiographic patterns of osteoarthritis of the knee joint in the community: The importance of the patellofemoral joint. *Ann Rheum Dis* 1992;51:844-849.
4. Barrett JP, Rashkoff E, Sirna EC, et al: Correlation of roentgenographic patterns and clinical manifestations of symptomatic idiopathic osteoarthritis of the knee. *Clin Orthop* 1990;253:179-183.
5. Oberlander MA, Baker CL, Morgan BE: Patellofemoral arthrosis: The treatment options. *Am J Orthop* 1998;27:263-270.
6. Tauton JE, Wilkinson M: Diagnosis and management of anterior knee pain. *Can Med Assoc J* 2001;164:1596-1601.
7. Boegard TL, Rudling O, Petersson IF, et al: Distribution of MR detected cartilage defects of the patellofemoral joint in chronic knee pain. *Osteoarthritis Cartilage* 2003;11:494-498.
8. Johnson LL, van Dyk GE, Green JR III, et al: Clinical assessment of asymptomatic knees: Comparison of men and women. *Arthroscopy* 1998;14:347-359.
9. Merchant AC: Patellofemoral imaging. *Clin Orthop* 2001;389:15-21.
10. Aglietti P, Buzzi R, Insall JN: Disorders of the patellofemoral joint, in Insall JN (ed): *Surgery of the Knee*, ed 2. New York, NY, Churchill Livingstone, 1993, pp 241-386.
11. Bullek DD, Kelly MA: Nonoperative treatment of patellofemoral pain, in Scott WN (ed): *The Knee*. St Louis, MO, Mosby-Year Book, 1994, pp 415-440.
12. Chrisman OD: The role of articular cartilage in patellofemoral pain. *Orthop Clin North Am* 1986;17:231-234.
13. Shoji H, Granada JL: Acid hydrolases in the articular cartilage of the patella. *Clin Orthop* 1974;99:293-297.
14. Ogilvie-Harris DJ, Jackson RW: The arthroscopic treatment of chondromalacia patellae. *J Bone Joint Surg Br* 1984;66:660-665.
15. Federico DJ, Reider B: Results of isolated patellar debridement for patellofemoral pain in patients with normal patellar alignment. *Am J Sports Med* 1997;25:663-669.
16. Schonholtz GJ, Ling B: Arthroscopic chondroplasty of the patella. *Arthroscopy* 1985;1:92-96.
17. Shneider D: Arthroscopy and arthroscopic surgery in patellar problems. *Orthop Clin North Am* 1982;13:407-413.
18. Pridie KH: A method of resurfacing osteoarthritic knee joints. *J Bone Joint Surg Br* 1959;41:618-619.
19. Zorman D, Prezerowitz L, Pasteels JL, et al: Arthroscopic treatment of posttraumatic chondromalacia patellae. *Orthopedics* 1990;13:585-588.
20. Bentley G: The surgical treatment of chondromalacia patella. *J Bone Joint Surg Br* 1978;60:74-81.
21. McCarroll JR, O'Donoghue DH, Grana WA: The surgical treatment of chrondromalacia of the patella. *Clin Orthop* 1983;175:130-134.
22. Childers JC Jr, Ellwood SC: Partial chondrectomy and subchondral bone drilling for chondromalacia. *Clin Orthop* 1979;144:114-120.
23. Hayes WC, Huberti HH, Lewallen DG, et al: Patellofemoral contact pressures and the effects of surgical reconstructive procedures, in Ewing JW (ed): *Articular Cartilage and Knee Joint Function: Basic Science and Arthroscopy*. New York, NY, Raven Press, 1990.
24. Galloway MT, Noyes FR: Cystic degeneration of the patella after chondroplasty and subchondral bone perforation. *Arthroscopy* 1992;8:366-369.
25. Jackson RW, Kunkel SS, Taylor GJ: Lateral retinacular release for patellofemoral pain in the older patient. *Arthroscopy* 1991;7:283-286.
26. Ficat D, Ficat C, Bailleux A: Syndrome d'hyperpression externe de la rotule (shpe): Son interet pour la connaissance de l'arthrose. *Rev Chir Orthop Reparatrice Appar Mot* 1975;61:39-59.
27. Cushner FD, Scott WN: Arthroscopic examination and treatment of the patellofemoral joint, in Scuderi GR (ed): *The Patella*. New York, NY, Springer-Verlag, 1995, pp 201-221.
28. Kolowich PA, Paulos LE, Rosenberg TD, et al: Lateral release of the patella: Indications and contraindications. *Am J Sports Med* 1990;18:359-365.
29. Johnson DP, Wakeley C: Reconstruction of the lateral patellar retinaculum following lateral release: A case report. *Knee Surg Sport Traum Arthrosc* 2002;10:361-363.
30. Aderinto J, Cobb AG: Lateral release for patellofemoral arthritis. *Arthroscopy* 2002;18:399-403.
31. Dzioba RB: Diagnostic arthroscopy and longitudinal open lateral release: A four year follow up study to determine

predictors of surgical outcome. *Am J Sports Med* 1990;18: 343-348.

32. Aglietti P, Pisaneschi A, Buzzi R, et al: Arthroscopic lateral release for patellar pain and instability. *Arthroscopy* 1989; 5:176-183.

33. Scuderi GR, Cuomo F, Scott WN: Lateral release and proximal realignment for patella subluxation and dislocation: A long term follow up. *J Bone Joint Surg Am* 1988;70: 856-861.

34. Maquet P: Un traitement biomecanique de l'arthrose femero-patellaire. *Rev Rheum Mal Osteoartic* 1963;30: 779-783.

35. Maquet P: Mechanics and osteoarthritis of the patellofemoral joint. *Clin Orthop* 1979;144:70-73.

36. Bandi W: Chondromalacia patellae and femoropatellar arthrosis. *Helv Chir Acta* 1972;1:3.

37. Fulkerson JP: *Disorders of the Patellofemoral Joint.* Baltimore, MD, Williams & Wilkins, 1996.

38. Ferguson AB, Brown TD, Fu FH, et al: Relief of patellofemoral contact stress by anterior displacement of the tibial tubercle. *J Bone Joint Surg Am* 1979;61:159-166.

39. Nakamura N, Ellis M, Seedhom BB: Advancement of the tibial tubercle: Biomechanical studies. *J Bone Joint Surg Br* 1985;67:255-260.

40. Fernandez L, Usabaga J, Yubero J, et al: An experimental study of the redistribution of patellofemoral pressure by the anterior displacement of the anterior tuberosity of the tibia. *Clin Orthop* 1989;238:183-194.

41. Fulkerson JP, Becker GJ, Meaney JA, et al: Anteromedial tibial tubercle transfer without bone graft. *Am J Sports Med* 1990;18:490-497.

42. Radin EL: The Maquet procedure: Anterior displacement of the tibial tubercle: Indications, contraindications, and precautions. *Clin Orthop* 1986;213:241-248.

43. Rappoport LH, Browne MG, Wickiewicz TL: The Maquet osteotomy. *Orthop Clin North Am* 1992;23:645-656.

44. Maquet P: Advancement of the tibial tuberosity. *Clin Orthop* 1976;115:225-230.

45. Jenny JY, Sader Z, Henry A, et al: Elevation of the tibial tubercle for patellofemoral pain syndrome: An 8 to 15 year follow up. *Knee Surg Sport Traum Arthrosc* 1996;4: 92-96.

46. Radin EL, Pan HQ: Long term follow up study on the Maquet procedure with special reference to the causes of failure. *Clin Orthop* 1993;290:253-258.

47. Mendes DG, Soudry M, Iusim M: Clinical assessment of Maquet tibial tuberosity advancement. *Clin Orthop* 1987; 222:228-238.

48. Ferguson AB: Elevation of the insertion of the patellar ligament for patellofemoral pain. *J Bone Joint Surg Am* 1982; 64:766-771.

49. Bessette GC, Hunter RE: The Maquet procedure: A retrospective review. *Clin Orthop* 1988;232:159-167.

50. Putz P, Mokassa L, Janssens JL, et al: Tibial fractures following Maquet's tuberosity advancement. *Acta Orthop Belgica* 1990;56:477-481.

51. Fulkerson JP: Anteromedialization of the tibial tubercle for patellofemoral malalignment. *Clin Orthop* 1983;177: 176-181.

52. Fulkerson JP: Technique of lateral retinacular release and anteromedial tibial tubercle transfer, in Harner CD, Vince KG, Fu FH (eds): *Techniques in Knee Surgery.* Philadelphia, PA, Lippincott Williams & Wilkins, 2001, pp 123-129.

53. Morshuis WJ, Pavlov PW, DeRooy KP: Anteromedialization of the tibial tubercle in the treatment of patellofemoral pain and malalignment. *Clin Orthop* 1990;255:242-250.

54. Post WR, Fulkerson JP: Distal realignment of the patellofemoral joint: Indications, effects, results, and recommendations. *Orthop Clin North Am* 1992;23:631-643.

55. Cosgarea AJ, Freedman JA, McFarland EG: Nonunion of the tibial tubercle shingle following Fulkerson osteotomy. *Am J Knee Surg* 2001;14:51-54.

56. Godde S, Rupp S, Dienst M, et al: Fracture of the proximal tibia six months after Fulkerson osteotomy: A report of two cases. *J Bone Joint Surg Br* 2001;83:832-833.

57. Diduch DR, Insall JN, Scott WN, et al: Total knee replacement in young active patients: Long term follow up and functional outcome. *J Bone Joint Surg Am* 1997;79:575-582.

58. Hoffman AA, Heithoff SM, Camargo M: Cementless total knee arthroplasty in patients 50 years or younger. *Clin Orthop* 2002;404:102-107.

59. Rand JA, Trousdale RT, Ilstrup DM, et al: Factors affecting the durability of primary total knee prostheses. *J Bone Joint Surg Am* 2003;85:259-265.

60. Hsu HC, Luo ZP, Rand JA, et al: Influence of patellar thickness on patellar tracking and patellofemoral contact characteristics after total knee arthroplasty. *J Arthroplasty* 1996;11:69-80.

61. Kelly MA: Patellofemoral complications following total knee arthroplasty. *Inst Course Lect* 2001;50:403-407.

62. Cartier P, Sanouiler JL, Grelsamer R: Patellofemoral arthroplasty: Two to 12 year follow up study. *J Arthroplasty* 1990;5:49-55.

63. McKeever DC: Patellar prosthesis. *J Bone Joint Surg Am* 1955;37:1074-1084.

64. Depalma AF, Sawyer B, Hoffman JD: Reconsiderations of lesions affecting the patellofemoral joint. *Clin Orthop* 1962;18:63-85.

65. Levitt RL: A long term evaluation of patellar prosthesis. *Clin Orthop* 1973;97:153-157.

66. Insall JN, Tria AJ, Aglietti P: Resurfacing of the patella. *J Bone Joint Surg Am* 1980;62:933-936.

67. Harrington KD: Long term results for the McKeever patellar resurfacing prosthesis used as a salvage procedure for severe chondromalacia patellae. *Clin Orthop* 1992;279: 201-213.

68. Kooijman HJ, Driessen AP, van Horn JR: Long-term results of patellofemoral arthroplasty: A report of 56 arthroplasties with 17 years follow up. *J Bone Joint Surg Am* 2003;85:336-340.

69. Tauro B, Ackroyd CE, Newman JH, et al: The Lubinus patellofemoral arthroplasty: A five to ten year prospective study. *J Bone Joint Surg Br* 2001;83:696-701.

70. Ackroyd CE, Newman JH, Webb JM: Abstract: The Avon patello-femoral arthroplasty: Two to five year results. *70ᵗʰ Annual Meeting,* Rosemont, IL, American Academy of Orthopaedic Surgeons.

71. Ackroyd CE, Polyzoides AJ: Patellectomy for osteoarthritis: A study of 81 patients followed from two to twenty-two years. *J Bone Joint Surg Br* 1970;60:353-357.

72. Brittberg M, Lindahl A, Nilsson A, et al: Treatment of full thickness cartilage defects in human knee with cultured autologous chondrocytes. *N Engl J Med* 1994;331:889-895.

73. Laskin RS, van Stejin M: Total knee replacement for patients with patellofemoral arthritis. *Clin Orthop* 1999; 367:89-95.

74. Parvizi J, Stuart MJ, Pagnano MW, Hanssen AD: Total knee arthroplasty in patients with isolated patellofemoral arthritis. *Clin Orthop* 2001;392:147-152.

75. Lynch AF, Rorabeck CH, Bourne RB: Extensor mechanism complications following total knee arthroplasty. *J Arthroplasty* 1987;2:135-140.

76. Scuderi GR, Insall JN, Scott WN: Patellofemoral pain after total knee arthroplasty. *J Am Acad Orthop Surg* 1994;2: 239-246.

77. Healy WL, Wasilewski SA, Takei R, et al: Patellofemoral complications following total knee arthroplasty: Correlation with implant design and patient risk factors. *J Arthroplasty* 1995;10:197-201.

78. Miller MC, Berger RA, Petrella AJ, et al: Optimizing femoral component rotation in total knee arthroplasty. *Clin Orthop* 2001;392:38-45.

79. Kawano T, Miura H, Nagamine R, et al: Factors affecting patellar tracking after total knee arthroplasty. *J Arthroplasty* 2002;17:942-947.

80. Poilvache PL, Insall JN, Scuderi GR, et al. Rotational landmarks and sizing of the distal femur in total knee arthroplasty. *Clin Orthop* 1996;331:35-46.

81. Greenfield MA, Insall JN, Case GC, et al: Instrumentation of the patellar osteotomy in total knee arthroplasty: The relationship of patellar thickness and lateral retinacular release. *Am J Knee Surg* 1996;9:129-131.

82. Gunal I, Karatosun V: Patellectomy: An overview with reconstructive procedures. *Clin Orthop* 2001;389:74-78.

83. Kelly MA, Brittis DA: Patellectomy. *Orthop Clin North Am* 1992;23:657-663.

84. Gunal I, Taymaz A, Kose N, et al: Patellectomy with vastus medialis obliqus advancement for comminuted patellar fractures: A prospective randomized trial. *J Bone Joint Surg Br* 1996;78:13-16.

85. Compere CL, Hill JA, Lewinnek GE, et al: A new method of patellectomy for patellofemoral arthritis. *J Bone Joint Surg Am* 1979;61:714-719.

86. Boucher HH: Results of excision of the patella. *J Bone Joint Surg Br* 1952;34:516-521.

87. Ackroyd CE, Polyzoides AJ: Patellectomy for osteoarthritis. *J Bone Joint Surg Br* 1978;60:353-357.

88. Kelly MA, Insall JN: Patellectomy. *Orthop Clin North Am* 1986;17:289-295.

89. Lennox IA, Cobb AG, Knowles J, et al: Knee function after patellectomy: A 12 to 48 year follow up. *J Bone Joint Surg Br* 1994;76:485-487.

90. Feller JA, Bartlett RJ: Patellectomy and osteoarthritis: Arthroscopic findings following previous patellectomy. *Knee Surg Sport Traum Arthrosc* 1993;1:159-161.

CHAPTER 9

PATELLOFEMORAL ARTICULAR CARTILAGE TREATMENT

JACK FARR, MD

Because of the unique qualities of the patellofemoral joint, articular cartilage lesions of this joint cannot be best treated by simply applying treatment algorithms used for tibiofemoral articular cartilage lesions. Brittberg and associates[1] brought attention to this critical point when they reported on clinical outcomes of autologous cultured chondrocyte transplantation that showed a high percentage of good or excellent results at the tibiofemoral joint and a high percentage of fair or poor results at the patellofemoral joint. In a later study, the approach was altered to concomitantly address specific balance, load, contact area, and alignment pathologies at the time of or preceding articular cartilage restoration, and outcomes improved markedly.[2] [Note: Use of autologous cultured chondrocytes is "off-label" at the patella and "on-label" at the trochlea in regards to FDA package insert instructions.] These findings demonstrate the importance of adhering to underlying patellofemoral management concepts when applying cartilage restoration techniques. It must also be kept in mind that patellofemoral surgery can affect the articular cartilage. For example, the historic Hauser procedure was considered an acceptable patellofemoral surgical technique because it successfully prevented recurrent patellar instability; however, articular cartilage overload occurred as a result of a posteriorization component during medialization of the tibial tubercle. The increased patellofemoral stress led to gradual patellofemoral articular cartilage deterioration.[3] The outcomes of the various treatment options discussed in this chapter are influenced tremendously by patient factors, many of which the surgeon has little control over. Minas (T Minas, MD, Toronto, Canada, unpublished data, 2002) reported that a patient's preoperative general perception of his or her quality of life as measured by the Medical Outcomes Study 36-Item Short Form Health Survey is more predictive of outcome score than is the position or size of the articular cartilage lesion. As biologic factors play out potentially months after restorative surgery, it becomes apparent that patellofemoral cartilage restoration outcomes are also dependent on patient compliance with specific instructions regarding weight bearing, range of motion, and rehabilitation.

The fact that articular cartilage does not contain nerve fibers complicates the attempt to assign a component of a patient's patellofemoral pain to patellofemoral cartilage lesions. Pain, being a central brain perception of peripheral nerve stimulation, is very complex. The central brain connection and influence must be considered when evaluating variable patient responses to the same treatment. This reinforces the finding that not all outcomes are based solely on the local response to treatment. Several authors have studied the basis of patellofemoral pain. Ficat and Hungerford[4] reported on the contribution of elevated intraosseous pressures. Although there are multiple hypotheses as to the cause of elevated patellofemoral intraosseous pressures, recent studies on the overloading phenomenon as it relates to articular cartilage lesions show an increase in stress levels in the cartilage around the lesions (shoulder area or cartilage rim stress) in defects that are larger than 1 cm in diameter.[5] Other suggested sources of pain exacerbated by patellar chondrosis include the capsule, patellofemoral soft-tissue constraints, and synovium, all of which may be irritated by chondral debris that activates an inflammatory/nociceptive small molecule cascade. On the other hand, many patients with patellofemoral pain have intact articular cartilage, and occasionally patients with "bone on bone" patellofemoral joints with associated chronic patellar subluxation report only stiffness and occasional aching. Even after considering all other factors, a group of patients will remain with patellofemoral pain that is caused by a cartilage lesion. Such patellofemoral cartilage lesions are the topic of this chapter.[6]

When patellofemoral treatment is contemplated, the effect on the patellofemoral joint biomechanics and the articular cartilage may be considered separately initally to simplify the process. After these separate algorithms suggest management options, they are then reconsidered within the framework of the very unique features involving patellofemoral joint articular cartilage lesions and the patellofemoral pain patient.

Articular cartilage lesions usually have a multifactorial etiology; therefore, this chapter first considers the classification of the cartilage lesion and then examines it in the context of the patellofemoral joint. Similarities and differences between patellofemoral and tibiofemoral cartilage lesions are evaluated, as well as how tibiofemoral cartilage treatment is modified when its effect on the patellofemoral joint is considered.

BASIC SCIENCE OF PATELLOFEMORAL CARTILAGE

An understanding of normal patellofemoral articular cartilage is necessary to appreciate its pathology and the goals of treatment. Articular cartilage in all joints is anisotropic; that is, it demonstrates position-specific composition of both the cellular and matrix components. This follows the body's efficiency of form following function. Some of the thickest cartilage is found at the patellofemoral joint because it is subjected to some of the highest loads in the body. As in other areas of the knee joint, convex areas are thicker than concave areas. Bony morphology varies from the normal-appearing articulation, with highly contained and congruent patellofemoral joint surfaces, to the extremely dysplastic patella and trochlea, where the patella is essentially flat and the trochlea is convex. These factors are important, not only in osteochondral transfer or transplant matching but also in cell therapy because they affect the time required for the reestablishment of a full-thickness construct. In addition, Staubli and associates[7] used MRI to demonstrate that the articular cartilage contour does not always match the bony contour (Fig. 1). This finding is very important in preoperative planning because reliance on bony radiographic landmarks only may cause the surgeon to create bony congruence that in fact is incompatible with the contour of the articular cartilage.

DESCRIPTION OF ARTICULAR CARTILAGE LESIONS

Classification

Most classifications of articular cartilage lesion have historic links to the 1961 article by Outerbridge.[8] However, the various modifications of the Outerbridge classification system have caused some confusion. The original article outlined a classification that combined both size and lesion appearance (fibrillation/fissuring) for type 2 (less than ½ inch in diameter) and type 3 (greater than ½ inch in diameter). Currently, most surgeons report chondrosis using three separate data points: (1) surface area of the lesion; (2) depth of the chondrosis (closed with no substance loss, open chondrosis to 50% of the depth of the surrounding cartilage, 50% of the depth to the level of bone, full-thickness loss with exposed bone, or full-thickness cartilage loss that also involves bony loss); and (3) position of the lesion. The International Cartilage Repair Society (ICRS) has developed both a position-reporting grid (Fig. 2) and a measure of depth that are available as part of the ICRS Cartilage Injury Evaluation Package on their website at www.cartilage.org.[9] The modified Outerbridge classification system used in the United States by many surgeons and the formal classifications of Noyes and Stabler[10] both differ from the ICRS, as shown in Table 1 and Figure 3.

FIGURE 1

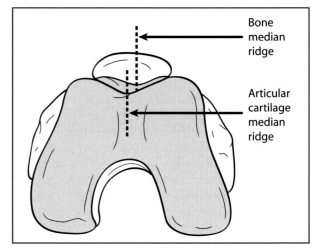

Mismatch of patellofemoral articular contour and bony contour.

FIGURE 2

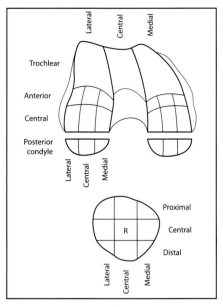

ICRS mapping grid scale for patellofemoral cartilage lesions.

FIGURE 3

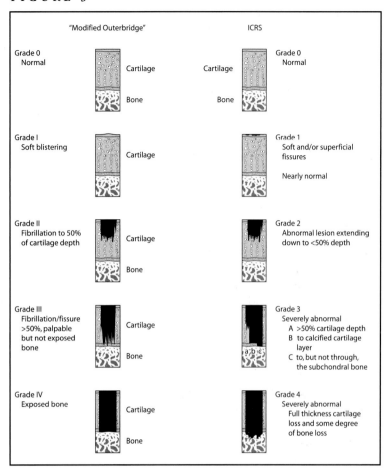

Comparison of the modified Outerbridge and ICRS classification systems.

Other Factors

In addition to the classification of the articular cartilage lesion, other factors, such as marginal osteophytes or the less frequently discussed intralesional osteophytes, may enter into the planning process for cartilage restoration (Fig. 4). The remaining cartilage surrounding the lesion ("shoulder the lesion") must be evaluated as to whether it contains the lesion (contained defect) or not (uncontained defect). Furthermore, initially appearing normal cartilage not directly involved with the lesion may not in fact be completely normal. Numerous genetic factors direct the composition of the cellular and the matrix components, thereby determining whether or not the remaining articular cartilage is predisposed to degeneration.[11] In addition, the apparently normal articular carti-lage may show a decreased chondrocyte population with age and changes occur in the composition of the matrix over time.[12] Volumetric MRI may be used to show articular cartilage attrition and further aid in making preoperative planning decisions.[13]

CATEGORIES OF PATELLOFEMORAL CHONDROSIS PRESENTATION

The goal of assigning certain patellofemoral cartilage presentations to specific subgroups is threefold: (1) to improve understanding of the pathology, (2) to help direct optimal treatment applications, and (3) to allow a logical analysis of the outcomes. This loop—defining treatment for specific subgroups followed by outcome

TABLE 1

Comparison of Classic Outerbridge, Modified Outerbridge, Noyes, and ICRS Articular Cartilage Classifications

	Classic Outerbridge	Modified Outerbridge	Noyes	ICRS
Grade 0		Normal		Normal
Grade 1	Softening	Softening	A. Softening with resilience B. Extensive softening	A. Near normal B. Soft intact or superficial open lesion
Grade 2	Fragmentation fissuring <1/2 in diameter	Open fissures, fibrillation to 50% depth	Open chondrosis A. <1/2 thickness of normal B. ≥1/2 thickness of normal	Abnormal lesion to < 50% cartilage depth
Grade 3	Fragmentation fissuring >1/2 in diameter	Open fissure fibrillation to palpable bone (>50% depth)	Exposed bone A. Bone surface intact B. Bone surface cavitation	Severely abnormal A. >50% cartilage depth B. Down to calcified layer C. To but not through bone
Grade 4	Erosion of cartilage down to bone	Exposed bone		Severely abnormal full-thickness cartilage loss and bone loss
Notes			Add diameter location and degree of knee flexion where the lesion is weight bearing	Add size (area) of lesion and site of lesion

analysis—allows continual improvements in understanding and patient treatment. Over the next few years, with improved understanding of the importance of underlying genetic factors for morphology and for articular cartilage grading, the addition of other classification subsets is certain to improve patient and surgical selection and understanding of the response to treatment. Only through critical assessment of patient outcomes can further refinements of the classifications lead to optimal treatment.

When developing subgroups for classifying patellofemoral cartilage lesions, information from the patellofemoral arthroplasty literature is useful because it is likely that many patellofemoral arthroplasty patients were candidates for cartilage restoration at some earlier point. Patellofemoral arthroplasties fail not only at the prosthesis but also by progression of tibiofemoral degenerative disease. This suggests two main subgroups of these patients: those with an underlying predisposition to articular cartilage degeneration and those with normal or

FIGURE 4

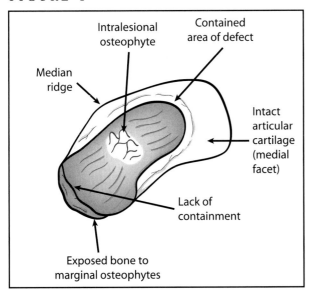

Additional descriptive factors of patellofemoral articular cartilage include intralesional osteophytes, marginal osteophytes, and containment.

near-normal articular cartilage. These groupings are useful for discussion, but until cartilage can be quality graded (by MRI, genetic assay, mechanical firmness testing, ultrasound composition estimates, etc), these groupings will remain a gross estimate. Currently, arthroscopic evaluation coupled with radiographic appearances (and, at times, with volumetric MRI cartilage data) can assist in assigning a patient to the group with patellofemoral cartilage deterioration associated with generalized joint deterioration or the group with apparent isolated patellofemoral chondrosis.

Patellofemoral Chondrosis With Associated Tibiofemoral Chondrosis

Patients with diffuse but predominantly patellofemoral chondrosis may have progression at a variable rate and failure at the tibiofemoral joint even after an initially "successful" patellofemoral arthroplasty. It is likely that tibiofemoral varus or valgus present at the time of the arthroplasty, not the patellofemoral arthroplasty, contributes most significantly to failure of the overloaded compartment. To slow progressive tibiofemoral chondrosis and ultimate failure, realignment of the tibiofemoral axis is recommended. In patients undergoing cartilage restoration, articular cartilage lesions on both the tibiofemoral and patellofemoral joints are common. To opti-

mize the outcome, both areas are treated, but it must be appreciated that this is a different subgroup than patients with isolated patellofemoral chondrosis and probably has a poorer prognosis. In addition, tibiofemoral forces change as patellofemoral alignment is changed and vice versa. For example, Kuroda and associates[14] have shown in the laboratory that tubercle medialization may increase medial tibiofemoral compartment loading.

Subsets within this group include patients with additional tibiofemoral considerations such as ligament and meniscal deficiencies that require advanced restoration considerations (eg, meniscal allograft transplantation, anterior cruciate ligament reconstruction) beyond the scope of this chapter. Also, patients with predominantly patellofemoral chondrosis and more generalized underlying chondrosis need to be counseled regarding future potential tibiofemoral treatments. Finally, in the older patient with predominantly "isolated" patellofemoral disease, some authors recommend patellofemoral arthroplasty and others recommend total joint arthroplasty. The ultimate goal of cartilage restoration is to restore the joint to avoid arthroplasty, but because of the limitations of biology in the older patient, if patellofemoral cartilage restoration is performed, the patient should be counseled thoroughly regarding realistic expectations.

Isolated Patellofemoral Chondrosis

Isolated patellofemoral chondrosis without tibiofemoral chondrosis (or a genetic propensity for the same) can be divided into the following categories: traumatic, dysplastic, and focal osteochondral defects. Overlap does occur, such as a dysplastic patellofemoral joint that sustains an osteochondral fracture during dislocation/reduction; however, the divisions help in determining the optimal treatment.

Traumatic Lesions

The traumatic group can be further subdivided into microtrauma and macrotrauma. Microtrauma includes repetitive overuse injuries and may include some cases of isolated trochlear chondrosis in a joint with normal alignment and morphology in patients involved with basketball, Alpine skiing, weight training, fencing, and other high patellofemoral loading activities. Macrotrauma involves either an episode of patellar instability or a direct impact. Patellar subluxation may create linear fissures in the patella, whereas frank dislocation may cause a medial facet chondral fracture (traumatic delamina-

FIGURE 5

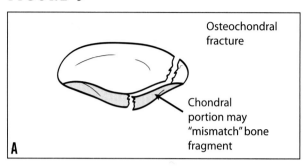

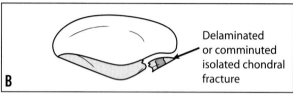

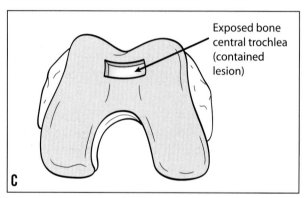

Types of isolated patellofemoral chondrosis. **A,** Medial facet osteochondral fracture. **B,** Medial facet chondral fracture. **C,** Overuse chondrosis of the central trochlea.

FIGURE 6

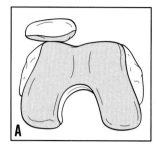 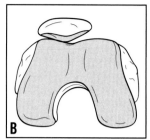

Two dysplastic examples with associated subluxation. **A,** More lateral position and shallower patella and trochlea. **B,** Less lateral position.

tion) or an osteochondral fracture injury (Fig. 5). Depending on the degree of knee flexion at the time of the injury, the femoral trauma may be at the lateral margin of the trochlea or, more commonly, the lateral margin of the lateral femoral condyle just distal to the level of the notch roof. In these latter injuries, occasionally the shear force injures a portion of the weight-bearing area of the lateral femoral condyle; therefore, tibiofemoral implications must be addressed. Osteochondral fractures can be repaired according to the standards of any joint fracture reduction and internal fixation. Chondral-only delaminating injuries often have a thin wisp of calcified cartilage/bone; these may also be repaired. For these injuries, chondral darts, bioabsorbable screws, or suturing to bone may be more optimal than pin/screw fixation used for standard osteochondral fragments. Irreducible or markedly comminuted fragments may require débridement, followed by consideration of future restoration options. In both of these situations, treatment of the underlying patellofemoral problem (eg, realignment and/or repair) is essential to avoid abnormal forces on any cartilage repair or restoration.

Dysplastic Lesions

The dysplastic group is quite heterogeneous (Fig. 6). Even the definition of dysplasia and/or malalignment allowing assignment of a patellofemoral joint to a particular subgroup is highly controversial. To be useful, the subgroup classifications must reflect the role of dysplasia in altering patellofemoral contact areas and thus stress. When the stress exceeds the margin of safety for a particular patient's articular cartilage, wear chondrosis appears. The quality of the underlying articular cartilage also varies, resulting in different rates of chondrosis progression among individuals with similar-appearing dysplasias. The margin of safety for articular cartilage is relatively small at the patellofemoral joint, partly because of the high forces and small contact areas even in the normal knee.

Dysplastic patellofemoral joints are currently treated by adjusting the soft tissues (proximal surgery) and attachment points (distal or tubercle surgery) (Fig. 7, A and B). Controversy remains regarding altering the patellofemoral morphology (trochleoplasty and patelloplasty) (Fig. 7, C). From an articular cartilage standpoint, it is important to strive to improve the contact area and decrease force (eg, anteromedialization for lateral patellar and/or trochlear chondrosis at the time of cartilage restoration), thus decreasing stress (force per unit area) to the restoration tissue. Likewise, it is important not to overconstrain the joint, such as with overly aggressive

FIGURE 7

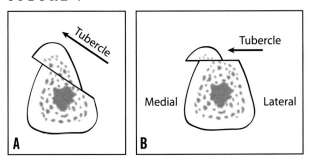

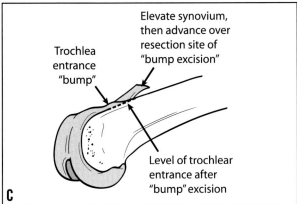

A, Fulkerson anteromedialization. B, Elmslie-Trillat medialization. C, Peterson trochleoplasty.

FIGURE 8

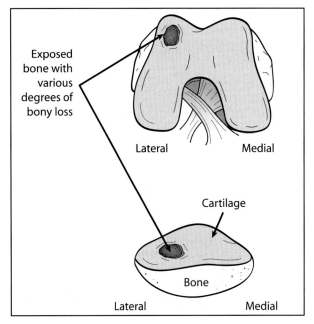

Osteochondritis of the central patella and lateral trochlea.

nonphysiologic medial reefing. In obese patients, these biomechanic overloads are confounded with an excessive body mass index. Because of the multifactorial nature of patellofemoral chondrosis, it is difficult to define a specific weight limit, but certainly there exists some limit over which any cartilage restoration will fail. Therefore, caution and extensive counseling are advised. For most activities of daily living on level ground, however, the patellofemoral joint is subjected to less than 50% of body weight, allowing for modification of activity to decrease loads to the patellofemoral joint to an acceptable level in some marginal patients who are overweight but not severely obese.

Focal Osteochondral Lesions
The third group includes focal osteochondral lesions associated with an underlying focal bony necrosis (Fig. 8). Although relatively rare at the patellofemoral joint, both osteonecrosis and osteochondritis dissecans do occur, sometimes in otherwise normal joints. Osteochondritis dissecans lesions of the patellofemoral joint are most like-

ly related to some type of repetitive overload with an underlying genetic predisposition that causes a focal area of bone to die with normal overlying articular cartilage. These lesions are managed with the same algorithm as for tibiofemoral osteochondritis dissecans with the exception of observing patellofemoral-specific management to optimize the contact area and minimize force. Osteonecrosis may have a more systemic underlying etiology. Once predisposing factors are addressed and the lesion has become quiescent (burned out), it may be addressed the same as other focal areas of osteochondral pathology, with the understanding that bony management is as important as chondral treatment. During the bony treatment, extra effort should be made to ensure that all dead and marginal bone is removed before beginning the restorative portion of the procedure. This may involve staging: first, a deep cancellous bone grafting, and later, cartilage restoration. Without a healthy bone base, cartilage treatment is at high risk for failure.

CARTILAGE RESTORATION OPTIONS

Cartilage restoration options for the patellofemoral joint parallel those for the tibiofemoral joint with certain modifications in technique and postoperative weight bearing, range of motion, and rehabilitation. There is a broad array of techniques, with large areas of overlap in application. The "demand match" approach developed by arthroplasty surgeons—in which the demand a patient is expected to place on an implant is considered when selecting the implants—was adapted to biologic restoration through a treatment algorithm for cartilage restoration. Patient-specific factors include activity level, physiologic age, and, in the future, possibly the quality of the noninvolved articular cartilage. General knee-specific factors include meniscal function status, alignment, and ligament status; patellofemoral status is classified as discussed earlier. Cartilage-specific technique considerations include cost, primary versus salvage, availability of technology, and lesion-specific parameters (surface dimensions, depth, and containment). These guidelines, when applied to the patellofemoral joint, must also consider the probability of a successful outcome from the patient's perspective. Once again, a patellofemoral-specific plan of treatment is formulated. If chondrosis is present, a staged versus concomitant approach may be taken.

To illustrate the combining of patellofemoral and cartilage restoration algorithms, consider a patient with patellofemoral dysplasia who has chronic lateral positioning of the patella relative to the central sulcus and lateral patellar tilt. Distally, there is an increase from normal in the lateral distance of the tibial tubercle to the sulcus midpoint. The patient does not have patellar instability. The question of whether patellofemoral joint chondrosis is present is difficult to determine preoperatively. If nonsurgical treatment fails to provide relief, tibial tubercle medialization, which includes lateral release as appropriate, is considered. From a strictly patellofemoral viewpoint, this knee is a Fulkerson classification II (subluxation and tilt). Before considering cartilage restoration options, treatment would typically consist of tibial tubercle medialization along a flat coronal plane (Elmslie-Trillat procedure) if there is minimal chondrosis, or anteromedialization if there is chondrosis predominantly of the lateral patella (Fig. 7, *A* and *B*). Note that trochlear involvement is predictive of a limited positive outcome, and proximal or medial chondrosis suggests a very guarded outcome. If cartilage restoration options are available, the treatment of grade 0, 1, or 2 chondrosis would not involve cartilage restoration, whereas grade 3 or 4 chondrosis would be considered for articular cartilage restoration either at the time of the realignment surgery or after

the isolated realignment surgery has yielded a less than optimal outcome. This example may serve as a reference during discussion of the options available for cartilage restoration in the next section.

Historic Biologic Restoration Treatments

It is beyond the scope of this chapter to present all the historic stepping-stones that have been important during the development of the biologic approach to the patellofemoral joint. Many of the early open procedures have been gradually adapted and now appear in another form, such as the Pridie technique of débridement that now falls in the category of marrow stimulation.[15] Other earlier patellofemoral techniques, such as interpositional arthroplasty, have not recently been advocated at the patellofemoral joint; however, it is possible that this historic technique may be reinvented with a new material/technique. Scapinelli and associates[16] conducted an extensive review of past and current techniques.

Current Trends in Patellofemoral Cartilage Restoration

Débridement and Lavage

Débridement and lavage are not truly restorative but are listed here as part of the spectrum of treatment options. In many human biologic systems, there are wide variations of response to any treatment, and the placebo effect exists to some extent in the treatment of cartilage and patellofemoral disease. Many cartilage restoration studies compare pretreatment scores with posttreatment scores without reference to a control group. Early studies suggested the beneficial effect of débridement and lavage for knee chondrosis, usually termed arthrosis. The positive attributes of débridement and lavage include removal of debris inciting mechanical and chemically mediated irritation. Although it did not address the patellofemoral joint (or the moderate amount of chondrosis typically under consideration for cartilage restoration), a controversial study that attempted to address the placebo effect recently questioned the efficacy of débridement and lavage.[17] Nevertheless, biologic cartilage restoration treatments must exceed the results of baseline standard isolated patellofemoral management to be scientifically accepted.

Although not originally designed to address the question of cartilage restoration outcomes, the work of Pidoriano and associates[18] and others treating patellofemoral chondrosis with realignment/elevation and débridement and lavage but without cartilage restoration may serve as historic comparison. That is, many patients with patellofemoral chondrosis in the past were quite satisfied initally with results of anteromedialization alone. Cartilage restoration must exceed either the outcome scores of these patients or exceed the durability/duration of this standard. Most outcome tools that measure patient satisfaction stress pain and function, however, and these alone may not be the best measurements for the final success of cartilage restoration. In the future, articular cartilage status may be included as a portion of the outcome. One example would be a patient who undergoes a distal Hauser realignment that results in the absence of pain and full function without instability; however, chondrosis then develops over a 10-year period. This patient should not be labeled a success. In another forward-looking example, two identically appearing patellofemoral joints with subluxation and chondrosis may be treated in different ways if the concept of demand match is applied. A 50-year-old patient may do well with anteromedialization alone for 15 years and then undergo a patellofemoral or total knee arthroplasty at age 65 years. Conversely, a 20-year-old patient with the same knee may best be treated with cartilage restoration with hope to avoid endoprosthetic arthroplasty at age 35 years.

Marrow Stimulation

Marrow stimulation is the global term for cartilage surgery, which is based on penetrating the subchondral plate to allow marrow cells to repopulate the cartilage defect and form fibrocartilage. This technique dates to the 1930s, when it was used in the hip by Pridie.[19] It was then extended to the knee in 1959. As open surgical techniques converted to arthroscopic techniques, numerous variations on marrow stimulation have been developed. The initial arthroscopic marrow stimulation technique, abrasion arthroplasty, is credited to Johnson[20] (Fig. 9). In 1997, Steadman and associates[21] introduced the microfracture technique of marrow stimulation. The results, which have usually been reported for all three compartments of the knee and not typically isolated to the patellofemoral joint, show the ingrowth of fibrocartilage and various extents of marginal integration. Fibrocartilage in other areas of the knee joint appears to function adequately in the near term, but it does not show the long-term durability of hyaline cartilage. Some studies suggest that outcomes are independent of the size of the lesion, but Gill[22] reported more pain at follow-up in patients with larger

lesions and no significant differences when comparing outcomes for patellofemoral lesions and tibiofemoral lesions. As referenced above, studies have shown minimal increases in the stress that occurs in the (apparently normal) articular cartilage shoulders of lesions up to 10 mm in diameter; therefore, there may be biomechanical support for use of this economical marrow stimulation management for smaller, well-shouldered lesions. Steadman and associates[21] attribute their superior results to strict adherence to a rehabilitation program, which requires minimal loading for 6 to 8 weeks and continuous passive motion. This strict regimen may produce an environment that creates a better quality of fibrocartilage. Future manipulation of the environment with genetic, molecular, electrophysical, and mechanical means may allow the pluripotential cells to undergo transformation into hyaline cartilage, allowing an expansion of applications.

Cell Therapy

Cell therapy, in the most inclusive sense, includes any cartilage restoration system using cells. This includes mar-

FIGURE 9

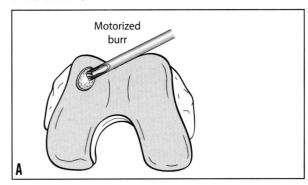

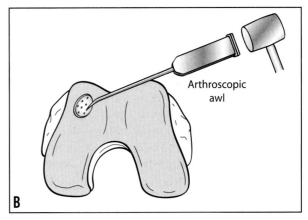

Abrasion arthroplasty (**A**) and microfracture (**B**).

row stimulation as well as pluripotential adult stem cells, embryonic stem cells, and allograft pluripotential cells. In this chapter, however, cell therapy is limited to autologous chondrocyte implantation (ACI), first popularized by Brittberg and associates.[23] The initial report of ACI retrospectively emphasized the importance of treating malpositioning of the patellofemoral joint; as in the original seven patellofemoral cases reported, only two had good or excellent results without correction of subluxation. Since that initial report, Brittberg and associates[23] reported patellofemoral ACI results that nearly mimic the results of the tibiofemoral compartments. Recently, in the United States, Minas (TM Minas, MD, personal communication, 2004) reviewed 45 patients who underwent patellofemoral ACI (off-label use per US Food and Drug Administration [FDA]-approved product labeling) and reported good and excellent results in 71%, fair results in 22%, and poor results in 7% with a 2- to 7-year follow-up. Note that in the United States, the only FDA-approved cultured chondrocyte application is a proprietary product, Carticel (Genzyme, Boston, MA), whereas in Europe several laboratories are producing cultured chondrocytes. At the time of FDA approval in 1997, the published work did not support use of Carticel in the patella. ACI is approved by the FDA for use at the femoral condyles and trochlea. With regard to the FDA-approved trochlear ACI use, review of the Carticel registry data demonstrates efficacy for isolated trochlear articular cartilage lesions at 4 years.[24]

ACI techniques have unique considerations at the patellofemoral joint. The patella and trochlea have complex topography, and special care must be used in applying the periosteal watertight patch to duplicate this shape and not create a flat appearance (Fig. 10). In addition, the patella and trochlea are often dysplastic and subluxated laterally with associated loss of containment laterally. To achieve a watertight seal, it may be possible to use bioabsorbable microanchors that, as with tibiofemoral lesions, are augmented with fibrin glue. The patellar cartilage is the thickest in the body; therefore, the volume of cell suspension indicated for a certain area will not at times completely fill the defect. Cell therapy is based on the surface area of the lesion; therefore, full volume fill is not necessary as long as the entire defect is coated with cells, often accomplished by "painting" the cells in the defect during delivery.

Cell therapy is rapidly evolving. In Europe, products are in research and clinical use that deliver cultured cells seeded into various parameters of a three-dimensional construct, obviating the need to harvest a periosteal patch and tediously suture it into place. Not all cell-culturing methods are the same, however, nor are the number, viability, and concentration of cells the same. Thus, the positive or negative results of one cultured chondrocyte system cannot be directly extrapolated to another system. For example, one product may use a scaffold composed of an ester of hyaluronic acid, another collagen, whereas others use a synthetic patch. Early outcomes appear to be in line with the now-classic Peterson ACI technique.[25] Regardless of the carrier, the goal is a less invasive and

FIGURE 10

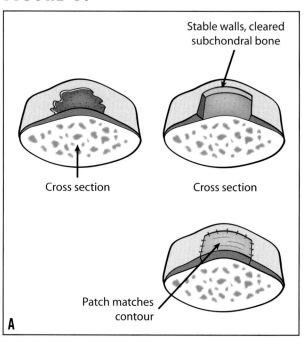

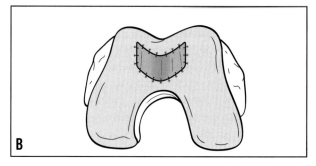

A, Patellofemoral cartilage lesion before and after débridement. **B,** Periosteal patch in place reproducing the contour of the patella and trochlea.

FIGURE 11

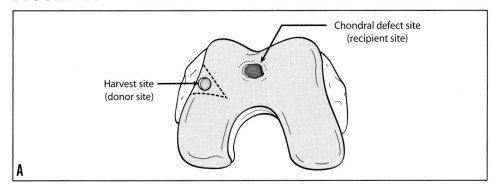

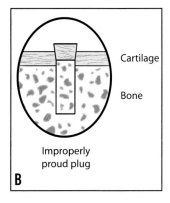

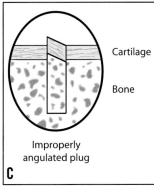

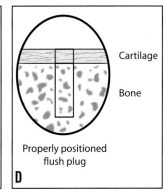

A, Harvest site of osteochondral plug. **B,** Improperly proud plug. **C,** Improperly angulated osteochondral plug. **D,** Properly positioned osteochondral plug.

technically less tedious procedure. Other novel cell delivery systems are under research and development. Key questions to ask when critically assessing any of these methods include: What happens to the implanted cells? (Mierisch and associates[26] explored this in a rabbit model.) How close to hyaline cartilage is the restored tissue biochemically and structurally (stratification of cells, extracellular matrix, and collagen network), and to what extent is there marginal and basilar (subchondral) integration?

Osteochondral Autograft

First popularized for use in the tibiofemoral joint by Bobic[27] and Hangody and associates,[28,29] small osteochondral cylindrical grafts have subsequently been used in the patellofemoral joint. Factors that play a role in applying osteochondral autografts in the patellofemoral joint include the challenge of matching the morphology of the harvest and recipient sites and the limited size of lesions to which this technique can be applied (Fig. 11). The typical osteochondral harvest sites are the trochlea/trochlear condylar junction and the notch. The notch morphology does not lend itself well to use in the patella or trochlea.

The trochlea/trochlear condylar intersection has limited tissue, and may be further limited when the site of pathology considered for treatment is near the same region. Bobic[27] reported that the typical maximal size of the defect that can be treated with this method is 1.5 cm², whereas Hangody and associates[28,29] do not share that limit. Lesions under 1.0 cm² are often asymptomatic, so this technique is applied to a somewhat narrow range of defect sizes. Regarding the various instrumentation sets to implement the technique, the subchondral bone of the patella is quite dense; therefore, it is more amenable to a drilling technique than a punch system. The goals are the same as in the tibiofemoral joint: a flush fit with a contour match. Patellar cartilage is considerably thicker than femoral articular cartilage thickness, however, so any femoral donor plug congruent at the surface will not be congruent at the tidemark. The effect of a donor plug surrounded by cartilage and not bone needs additional study. In the future, outcome studies of current implants will help refine the role for patellofemoral osteochondral plug transfer. These studies will also allow evaluation of the long-term effect of the harvest site.

Osteochondral Allograft

Osteochondral allograft has been available for many years. Frozen articular cartilage tissue did not offer long-term success because chondrocyte death resulted in gradual matrix breakdown, but implantation of fresh osteochondral allograft with viable chondrocytes produced intermediate-term results that made the procedure a reasonable option for patients with end-stage chondrosis. Aubin and associates[30] used this procedure in the knee. They reported excellent long-term results in patients with monopolar chondrosis, but its use in bipolar chondrosis produced markedly less promising results, and they discontinued its use. The patellofemoral joint has different loading patterns than the tibiofemoral joint, however, and it places the graft under different stress during remodeling. Chu and associates,[31] Meyers and associates,[32] and Bugbee[33] reported that the use of fresh patellofemoral osteochondral allografts in selected patients resulted in excellent pain relief and return of function at follow-up of more than 10 years. Unfortunately, because of concerns regarding transmission of infectious agents and bacterial graft infection, truly fresh

FIGURE 12

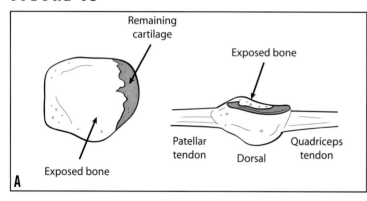

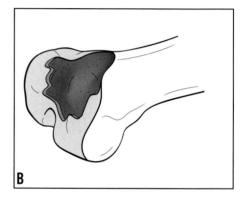

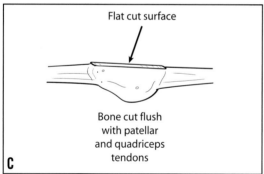

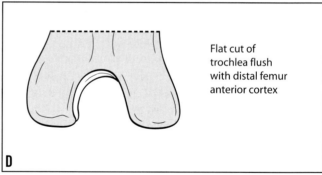

Flat cut of trochlea flush with distal femur anterior cortex

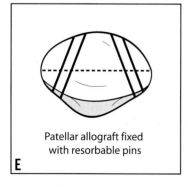

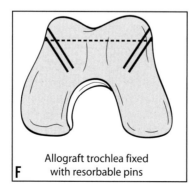

A, Patellar chondrosis. **B**, Trochlear chondrosis. **C**, Patellar cut. **D**, Trochlear cut. **E**, Transplanted patella. **F**, Transplanted trochlea.

allograft is no longer available in the United States. Allograft tissue is typically cooled in a culture medium while testing for safety of the graft is completed. Although such tissue is labeled "fresh," several studies have shown a gradual loss of chondrocyte viability over time.[34] The number of chondrocytes at a given time point during culturing varies (variables include time from harvest to cooling and culturing, number of cells at time zero, and culture medium); therefore, in light of the relatively hostile environment at the time of implant (hemarthrosis), osteochondral allografts should be implanted as soon as possible. Patellofemoral osteochondral allografts, typically used in patients with cartilage lesions, may push the limits of cell therapy treatment in terms of size, some degree of bone loss, and containment; therefore, the entire surface is usually replaced. Thus, rather than using the macro plugs often used in the tibiofemoral joint, the patella is often cut in the same manner as for patellofemoral arthroplasty and the trochlea is cut flat in a single plane exiting proximal to the notch roof (Fig. 12). Fixation is used to resist rotation and shear forces because compressive forces are inherent with the patellofemoral articulation. In addition to standard outside-in or inside-out screw interfragmentary fixation, it is possible to use resorbable pins, which have the advantage of less interference with future MRI evaluation or the need for removal with conversion to arthroplasty. In tibiofemoral allografts, size matching concomitantly matches the morphology (that is, similar-sized condyles have very similar morphology), whereas the morphology of the patellofemoral joint varies, even in knees the same size. This is not a problem if both the patella and trochlea are replaced, but if only one side is replaced, attempts should be made to match both size and morphology. In the postoperative period, the goals are to reestablish strength and motion and allow host transplant interface healing. After this initial healing, the patellofemoral joint is subject to creeping substitution; therefore, it is important to limit high loads to the joint. The patellofemoral joint experiences low loads during level ground walking but very high loads with stairs and inclines, so full weight bearing early may be allowed in the postoperative period, but stairs and inclines should be avoided for a prolonged period.

Bugbee (WD Bugbee, MD, Gothenberg, Sweden, unpublished data, 2000) classified patients as antibody positive or negative. Patients who were antibody negative had better clinical results and, compared with the tibiofemoral monopolar osteochondral allografts, the patellofemoral allografts had a higher percentage of antibody-positive patients. Nevertheless, in the relatively few total number of patients reported on, overall patellofemoral allograft results to date have been satisfactory.

Applying the demand match approach, the same large bipolar patellofemoral chondral lesions that may suggest an off-label use of cell therapy for a young patient might suggest an osteochondral allograft in a patient in early middle age. (Certainly, this scenario might suggest a patellofemoral arthroplasty in the patient in late middle age.) Although the literature would suggest that using truly fresh osteochondral allograft is a viable alternative for extensive patellofemoral chondrosis, the results may not be the same when using the "fresh cultured" osteochondral allograft currently available. Reviews of series using these currently available tissues will be the final test.

CONCLUSIONS

Patellofemoral chondrosis is not uncommon in patients with patellofemoral disease. Treatment algorithms need to take into consideration the biomechanical and articular cartilage-specific variables that led to the development of the chondrosis. After classification of the chondrosis etiology and documentation of the size, grade, and location of the cartilage loss, a demand match approach is used that factors in patient, knee, and patellofemoral-specific requirements.[35]

Just as patients are unaware of their risk for chondrosis, surgeons are also currently unable to accurately assess a patient's genetic risk for chondrosis other than noting the family history. MRI is increasingly used to assess articular cartilage, and parameters are being defined for identifying articular cartilage at risk for deterioration (eg, decreased volume, subchondral edema).[36] In the near future, the baseline cartilage quality may be assessed by cartilage-specific genetic testing.[37] This would potentially allow identification of a genetic predisposition to chondral degeneration, not only further refining treatment of patients with generalized arthritis with maximal expression at the patellofemoral joint, but also predicting which patients with chronic patellar subluxation are at risk for degeneration. Taken one step further, this would allow the development of a preventative medicine approach to patellofemoral treatment. All of this requires careful analysis of the natural history of patellofemoral problems in general, as well as those specifically involving the articular cartilage. Patellofemoral surgery, with its associated altered forces and contact areas, always has the potential of affecting the articular cartilage. When articular cartilage grading and patellofemoral natural history are combined, the goal of patellofemoral cartilage surgery may change from restoration to prophylactically altering the biomechanics in an attempt to preserve the articular cartilage.

In analyzing future patellofemoral outcome reports, it is important to evaluate both the study end points as well as comparisons and/or control subjects for clinical relevance. End points for assessing outcomes, such as clinical outcomes (pain and function), findings from noninvasive studies to assess tissue repair (such as MRI, genetic, and protein testing), and long-term assessment of the articular cartilage status, need refinement. A pain-free patient with full function may appear to be a short-term success, but if progressive chondral deterioration ultimately results in endoprosthetic arthroplasty, something is wrong with the measure of success. Patellofemoral articular cartilage surgery may, in time, be evaluated with regard to its success in maintaining articular cartilage homeostasis, in addition to obviously important clinical end points of pain and function.

Finally, medicine, orthopaedics, and patellofemoral cartilage restoration surgery are not practiced in a vacuum but rather in a real world with rising health care costs and demands. With expensive new technologies, procedural cost-effectiveness analyses will need to be applied while developing appropriate treatment guidelines. Recent economic analysis of cartilage restoration in the knee has demonstrated the overall cost benefits that are not obvious if only the isolated procedural costs are listed.[38,39] This information is very important for physicians, as patient advocates, to use in educating the health care "payers." There are increasing insurance industry, societal, and governmental pressures to reduce short-term health care costs. These pressures must be tempered with long-term outcomes that justify the short-term costs. Preservation of articular cartilage function is important in achieving optimal patellofemoral results.

REFERENCES

1. Brittberg M, Lindahl A, Nilsson A, Ohlsson C, Isaksson O, Peterson L: Treatment of deep cartilage defects in the knee with autologous chondrocyte transplantation. *New Engl J Med* 1994;331:889-895.
2. Brittberg M, Peterson L, Sjogren-Jansson E, Tallheden T, Lindahl A: Articular cartilage engineering with autologous chondrocyte transplantation. *J Bone Joint Surg Am* 2003; 85:109-115.
3. Fulkerson J: *Disorders of the Patellofemoral Joint.* Baltimore, MD, Williams and Wilkins, 1997.
4. Ficat P, Hungerford D: *Disorders of the Patellofemoral Joint.* Baltimore, MD, Williams and Wilkins, 1977.
5. Guettler J, Jurist K, Demetropoulos C, Yang K: Osteochondral defects in the human knee: Influence of defect size on cartilage rim stress and load redistribution to adjacent cartilage. *69th Annual Meeting.* Rosemont, IL, American Academy of Orthopaedic Surgeons, 2002.
6. Fulkerson J: Articular cartilage lesions in patellofemoral pain patients, in Fulkerson J (ed): *Disorders of the Patellofemoral Joint.* Baltimore, MD, Williams and Wilkins, 1997, pp 225-274.
7. Staubli H, Durrenmatt U, et al: Anatomy and surface geometry of the patellofemoral joint in the axial plane. *J Bone Joint Surg Br* 1999;81:452-458.
8. Outerbridge R: The etiology of chondromalacia patellae. *J Bone Joint Surg Br* 1961;43:752-757.
9. International Cartilage Repair Society: ICRS Cartilage Injury Evaluation Package, 2002. Available at www.cartilage.org. Accessed November 17, 2004.
10. Noyes FR, Stabler CL: A system for grading articular cartilage lesions at arthroscopy. *Am J Sports Med* 1989;17:505-513.
11. Aigner T, Zien A, Hanish D, Zimmer R: Gene expression in chondrocytes assessed with use of microarrays. *J Bone Joint Surg Am* 2003;85:117-123.
12. Martin JA, Buckwalter JA: The role of chondrocyte senescence in the pathogenesis of osteoarthritis and in limiting cartilage repair. *J Bone Joint Surg Am* 2003;85:106-110.
13. Burstein D, Gray M: New MRI techniques for imaging cartilage. *J Bone Joint Surg Am* 2003;85:70-77.
14. Kuroda R, Kambie H, Valdevit A, Andrish JT: Articular cartilage contact pressure after tibial tuberosity transfer: A cadaveric study. *Am J Sports Med* 2001;29:403-409.
15. Pridie KH: A method of resurfacing osteoarthritic knee joints. *J Bone Joint Surg Br* 1959;41:618-619.
16. Scapinelli R, Aglietti P, Baldovin M, Giron F, Teitge R: Biologic resurfacing of the patella: Current status. *Clin Sports Med* 2002;21:547-573.
17. Mosely JB, O'Malley K, Peterson NJ, et al: A controlled trial of arthroscopic surgery for osteoarthritis of the knee. *J Fam Pract* 2002;51:813.
18. Pidoriano AJ, Weinstein RN, Buuck DA, Fulkerson JP: Correlation of patellar articular lesions with results from anteromedial tibial tubercle transfer. *Am J Sports Med* 1997; 25:533-537.
19. Pridie KH: A method of resurfacing osteoarthritic knee joints. *J Bone Joint Surg Br* 1959;41:618.
20. Johnson LL: Arthroscopic abrasion arthroplasty historical and pathologic perspective: Present status. *Arthroscopy* 1986;2:54-69.
21. Steadman JR, Rodkey WG, Singleton SR, Briggs KK: Microfracture technique for full-thickness chondral

defects: Technique and clinical results. *Oper Tech Orthop* 1997;7:300-307.

22. Gill TJ: The treatment of articular cartilage defect using microfracture and debridement. *Am J Knee Surg* 2000;13: 33-40.

23. Brittberg M, Peterson L, Sjogren-Jansson E, Tallheden T, Lindahl A: Articular cartilage engineering with autologous chondrocyte transplantation. *J Bone Joint Surg Am* 2003; 85:109-115.

24. Micheli LJ, Browne JE, Fu F, et al: Full thickness articular cartilage defects of the trochlea: Management with ACI. *69th Annual Meeting*. Rosemont, IL, American Academy of Orthopaedic Surgeons, 2002.

25. Marcacci M, Zaffagnini S, Kon E, Vascellari A: Second-generation ACI technique, in *Management of Osteoarthritis of the Knee: An International Consensus*. Rosemont, IL, American Academy of Orthopaedic Surgeons, 2003, pp 49-58.

26. Mierisch CM, Wilson HA, Turner MA, Milbrandt TA, et al: Chondrocyte transplantation into articular cartilage defects with use of calcium alginate: The fate of the cells. *J Bone Joint Surg Am* 2003;85:1757-1767.

27. Bobic V: Arthroscopy osteochondral autogenous graft transplantation in anterior cruciate ligament reconstruction: A preliminary report. *Knee Surg Sports Traumatol Arthrosc* 1996;3:262-264.

28. Hangody L, Kish G, Karpati Z, Eberhart R: Osteochondral plugs: Autogenous osteochondral mosaicplasty for the treatment of focal chondral osteochondral articular defects. *Oper Tech Orthop* 1997;7:312-322.

29. Hangody LK, Rathonyi G: Management of osteochondral defects: Mosaicplasty technique, in *Management of Osteo-arthritis of the Knee: An International Consensus*. Rosemont, IL, American Academy of Orthopaedic Surgeons, 2003, pp 41-48.

30. Aubin P, Cheah HK, Davis AM, Gross AE: Long-term follow-up of fresh femoral osteochondral allografts for post-traumatic knee defects. *Clin Orthop* 2001;391:318-327.

31. Chu CR, Convery R, Hakeson WH: Fresh osteochondral allografting of the femoral condyle. *Clin Orthop* 1991;273: 139-145.

32. Meyers MH, Akeson W, Convery FR: Resurfacing of the knee with fresh allograft. *Clin Orthop* 1994;303:33-37.

33. Bugbee WD: Fresh osteochondral allografts. *J Knee Surg* 2002;15:191-195.

34. Williams SK, Amiel D, Ball ST, et al: Prolonged storage effects on the articular cartilage of fresh human osteo-chondral allografts. *J Bone Joint Surg Am* 2003;85: 2111-2120.

35. Cole BJ, Farr J: Putting it all together. *Oper Tech Orthop* 2001;11:151-154.

36. Laasanen M, Toyras J, Vasara AI, et al: Mechano-acoustic diagnosis of cartilage degeneration and repair. *J Bone Joint Surg Am* 2003;85:78-84.

37. Aigner T, Zien A, Hanisch D, Zimmer R: Gene expression in chondrocytes assessed with use of microarrays. *J Bone Joint Surg Am* 2003;85:117-123.

38 Minas T: Chondrocyte implantation in the repair of chon-dral lesions of the knee: Economics and quality of life. *Am J Orthop* 1998;27:739-744.

39. Lindahl A, Brittberg M, Peterson L: Health economics ben-efits following autologous chondrocyte transplantation for patients with focal chondral lesions of the knee. *Knee Surg Sports Traumatol Arthrosc* 2001;9:358-363.

INDEX

Notes: Page numbers followed by f indicate figures.
Page numbers followed by t indicate tables.

A

ACL. *See* Anterior cruciate ligament (ACL), 44
Activities of daily living (ADLs), 5-6
Activity modification therapy, 25
Acute patellar dislocation, 35-41
    epidemiology-related issues, 35
    imaging techniques, 36-40, 36*f*
      CT, 37
      MRI, 36-40, 36*f*
      radiographs, 36
    pathoanatomy-related issues, 35-36, 35*f*-36*f*
      MPFLs, 35-36, 35*f*-36*f*, 38-40, 38*t*
      VMO, 35-36, 35*f*-36*f*, 38-39, 38*t*
    patient histories, 39-40
    physical examinations, 39-40
    predisposition-related issues, 36-37
    recommendations, 39-40
    reference resources, 40-41
    treatments, 37-39, 37*t*-38*t*
      nonsurgical, 37-38, 37*t*
      surgical, 38-39, 38*t*
ADLs. *See* Activities of daily living (ADLs), 5-6
Albee osteotomy, 51
All-arthroscopic proximal realignment, 30-31, 31*f*
Allografts (osteochondral), 95-97, 96*f*
AMZ guides, 67-68
Anteromedialization, 63-69, 63*t*, 64*f*, 65*t*, 66*f*-67*f*, 69*f*
Anterior cruciate ligament (ACL), 44
Anteriorization and anteromedialization, 14-15, 14*f*-15*f*
Anteromedial tubercle transfer, 77-78
Anti-inflammatory treatments, 6
Arthritis (patellofemoral) with malalignment, 57-71
    bony considerations, 57-59, 57*f*-59*f*
    combined distal and proximal realignment, 63
    distal realignment by medial tibial tubercle transfer, 60-63, 62*f*, 63*t*
    Elmslie-Trillat procedure, 61-63, 62*f*, 63*t*
    etiology-related issues, 57
    imaging techniques, 57-59, 57*f*, 59*f*, 62*f*, 64*f*, 67*f*

    CT, 57-61, 59*f*
    radiographs, 57*f*, 58-60, 67*f*
    patient histories, 60
    physical examinations, 60
    procedure selection criteria, 59-60
    reference resources, 69-71
    symptomatic arthrosis and anteromedialization, 63-69, 63*t*, 64*f*, 65*t*, 66*f*-67*f*, 69*f*
    tubercle malalignment, 57-59, 57*f*-59*f*
Arthritis-related issues, 73-84. *See also under individual topics*
    arthritis (patellofemoral) with malalignment, 57-71
    isolated patellofemoral arthritis without malalignment, 73-84
Arthroplasty, 8, 78-80
    patellar hemiarthroplasty, 78-79, 78*f*
    patellofemoral, 78-79
    total knee, 80, 80*f*
    unicompartmental, 8
Arthroscopic medial imbrication, 13
Arthroscopic peripatellar synovectomy, 7-8, 7*f*
Arthroscopic reconstruction, 29-33. *See also* Mild patellar instability (arthroscopic reconstruction)
Arthroscopically assisted proximal realignment, 30
Arthroscopy, 75
Arthrosis and anteromedialization, 63-69, 63*t*, 64*f*, 65*t*, 66*f*-67*f*, 69*f*
Articular cartilage lesions, 86-87, 89*f*
    classification systems, 86-87, 87*f*, 88*t*
    genetic factors, 87
    osteophytes (marginal and intralesional), 87
Articular cartilage treatments, 85-99
    chondrosis presentation categories, 87-90, 89*f*-91*f*, 93*f*-96*f*
      isolated patellofemoral chondrosis, 89-90
      lesions (dysplastic), 90, 90*f*-91*f*
      lesions (focal osteochondral), 90-91
      lesions (traumatic), 90
      patellofemoral chondrosis with associated tibiofemoral chondrosis, 88-89
    imaging techniques, 86-88, 96-98
      MRI, 86-88, 96-98
      radiographs, 86-87
    pathology-related issues, 86, 86*f*
    reference resources, 98-99
    treatments (surgical restoration options), 91-97
      allografts (osteochondral), 95-97, 96*f*

autografts (osteochondral), 94-95, 95*f*
cell therapy, 93-95, 94*f*
débridement and lavage, 92-97
demand match approach, 91-92
Elmslie-Trillat procedure, 92
marrow stimulation, 92-93, 93*f*
Articular injuries, 36-37
Articular lesions, 13
ATT-TG (anterior tibial tubercle-trochlear groove) distances, 59, 59*f*
Autografts (osteochondral), 94-95, 95*f*
Axial radiographs, 23-24, 24*f*

B
Balance and timing (lower extremity), 11-12
Biomechanical studies, 64-65
Biomechanics (patellar instability), 43-44
Bracing, 25

C
Capsular stability, 45
Cartilage (articular), 85-99. *See also* Articular cartilage treatments
Caton-Deschamps ratios, 37
Cell therapy, 93-95, 94*f*
Cerebral palsy, 50
Charcot-Marie-Tooth disease, 21
Chondromalacia, 19-20
Chondroplasty, 8
Chondrosis presentation categories, 87-90, 89*f*-91*f*, 93*f*-96*f*
isolated patellofemoral chondrosis, 89-90
lesions, 90-91. *See also* Lesions
dysplastic, 90, 90*f*-91*f*
focal osteochondral, 90-91
traumatic, 90
patellofemoral chondrosis with associated tibiofemoral chondrosis, 88-89
Collateral stability, 45
Combined distal and proximal realignment, 63
Computed tomography (CT), 22, 24, 26, 37, 43, 46, 52, 57-61, 59*f*, 74, 74*f*
Concave impaction lesions, 36
Cruciate stability, 45
CT (computed tomography), 22, 24, 26, 37, 43, 46, 52, 57-61, 59*f*, 74, 74*f*

D
Débridement and lavage, 75, 92-97
Demand match approach, 91-92, 97
Differential diagnoses, 19, 19*f*
Dislocation. *See also under individual topics*
acute patellar, 35-41

recurrent patellar, 43-55
Distal realignment, 32-33, 60-63, 62*f*, 63*t*
Dynamic *vs.* static factors (pathophysiology), 20
Dysplastic lesions, 90, 90*f*-91*f*

E
Elmslie-Trillat procedure, 32-33, 61-63, 62*f*, 63*t*, 92
Ely test, 45
Epidemiology-related issues, 35, 43
Etiology-related issues, 57
Examinations (physical). *See* Physical examinations

F
FDA (Food and Drug Administration), 85, 93-94
Focal osteochondral lesions, 90-91
Fresh cultured grafts, 97
Fulkerson anteromedial tubercle transfer, 77-78
Fulkerson-type osteotomies, 26
Function envelopes, 4*f*

G
Gomori trichrome staining, 20

H
Hemiarthroplasty (patellar), 78-79, 78*f*
Hill-Sachs lesions, 36
Historical perspectives, 1, 1*f*-2*f*
Histories. *See* Patient histories
Homeostasis (tissue), 1-9. *See also* Pain without malalignment (tissue homeostasis perspectives)
Hypermobility, 45

I
ICRS (International Cartilage Repair Society), 86-88, 87*f*, 88*t*
Imaging techniques. *See also under individual topics*
CT, 22, 24, 26, 37, 43, 46, 52, 57-61, 59*f*, 74, 74*f*
MRI, 2-5, 22, 24, 26, 29, 36-40, 36*f*, 43, 46, 52, 86-88, 96-98
radiographs, 23-24, 24*f*, 32*f*, 36, 46, 57*f*, 58-60, 67*f*, 73, 73*f*, 77*f*, 80*f*, 86-87
radionuclide imaging, 24
for specific disorders. *See also under individual disorders*
acute patellar dislocation, 36-40, 36*f*
arthritis (patellofemoral) with malalignment, 57-59, 57*f*, 59*f*, 62*f*, 64*f*, 67*f*
articular cartilage treatments, 86-88, 96-98
isolated patellofemoral arthritis without malalignment, 73-80
mild patellar instability (arthroscopic reconstruction), 29-33
pain without malalignment (tissue homeostasis perspectives), 2-7

recurrent patellar dislocation, 43-52
rotational malalignment (patella), 22-26, 23f-24f
technetium Tc 99m-MDP (methylene diphosphonate)
scintigraphy, 2-7
Imbrication (arthroscopic medial), 13
Instability (mild patellar), 29-33. *See also* Mild patellar
instability (arthroscopic reconstruction)
Intralesional osteophytes, 87
Isolated lateral retinacular release, 25
Isolated patellofemoral arthritis without malalignment, 73-84
imaging techniques, 73-80
CT, 74, 74f
radiographs, 73, 73f, 77f-78f, 80f
patient histories, 73-74
physical examinations, 73-74, 74f
reference resources, 81-84
treatments (nonsurgical), 74
treatments (surgical), 74-81
arthroplasty (patellofemoral), 78-79
arthroplasty (total knee), 80, 80f
arthroscopy, 75
débridement and lavage, 75
Fulkerson anteromedial tubercle transfer, 77-78
lateral release, 75-76
Maquet procedure, 76-77, 77f
patellar hemiarthroplasty, 78-79, 78f
patellectomy, 80-81
tibial tubercle elevation/osteotomy, 76-78, 77f
Isolated patellofemoral chondrosis, 89-90

J
J signs and j-tracking, 21, 48, 58-59, 59f

K
Knee functions, 2-4, 4f
Kneeing-in gaits, 45

L
Lateral dislocations, 35
Lateral patellofemoral angles (LPAs), 24
Lateral radiographs, 23, 24f
Lateral release, 13, 13f, 25, 30, 75-76
Lavage and débridement, 75, 92-97
Lesions, 13, 36, 86-91
ACLs, 86-87, 89f
articular, 13
concave impaction, 36
dysplastic, 90, 90f-91f
focal osteochondral, 90-91
Hill-Sachs, 36

intralesional osteophytes, 87
traumatic, 90
Ligaments. *See also under individual ligaments*
ACLs, 44
MPFLs, 13-15, 14f, 29, 35-36, 35f-36f, 38-40, 38t, 43-44, 48-52
Load restrictions, 6
Lower extremity balance and timing, 11-12
LPAs (lateral patellofemoral angles), 24
Lying prone, 45-46
Lying supine, 45

M
Magnetic resonance imaging (MRI), 2-5, 22, 24, 26, 29, 36-40,
36f, 43, 46, 52, 86-88, 96-98
Malalignment issues. *See also under individual topics*
arthritis (patellofemoral) with malalignment, 57-71
isolated patellofemoral arthritis without malalignment, 73-84
pain without malalignment (tissue homeostasis perspectives), 1-9
rotational malalignment (patella), 19-28
tubercle malalignment, 57-59
Mapping (neurosensory), 2f
Maquet procedure, 26, 32-33, 76-77, 77f
Marginal osteophytes, 87
Marrow stimulation, 92-93, 93, 93f
McConnell taping, 6
Medial patellofemoral ligaments (MPFLs), 13-15, 14f, 29, 35-36,
35f-36f, 38-40, 38t, 43-44, 48-52
Medial reefing, 30, 30f
Medial tibial tubercle transfer, 60-63, 62f, 63t
Medical Outcomes Study 36-Item Short Form Health Survey
(SF 36), 85
Midsubstance injuries, 36
Mild patellar instability (arthroscopic reconstruction), 29-33
imaging techniques, 29-33
MRI, 29
radiographs, 32f
MPFLs, 29
pathoanatomy-related issues, 29
reference resources, 33
treatments (surgical), 29-33
advantages, 29-30
all-arthroscopic proximal realignment, 30-31, 31f
arthroscopically assisted proximal realignment, 30
distal realignment, 32-33
Elmslie-Trillat procedure, 32-33
lateral release, 30
Maquet procedure, 32-33
medial reefing, 30, 30f
rehabilitation, 31
results, 31-32

Yamamoto technique, 30
Minimally invasive patellar realignment, 51
Miserable alignment syndrome, 44-45
Morton's neuroma, 20
Mosiacplasty, 66
Movie theater sign, 2, 6, 20
MPFLs (medial patellofemoral ligaments), 13-15, 14f, 29, 35-36, 35f-36f, 38-40, 38t, 43-44, 48-52
MRI (magnetic resonance imaging), 2-5, 22, 24, 26, 29, 36-40, 36f, 43, 46, 52, 86-88, 96-98
Multifocal injuries, 36
Multiple sclerosis, 21
Muscle strengthening (painless), 6

N

Natural history issues, 43
Neurosensory mapping, 2f
Nociceptive output, 3t
Nonsurgical treatments. *See also under individual topics*
 for acute patellar dislocation, 37-38, 37t
 for isolated patellofemoral arthritis without malalignment, 74
 for pain without malalignment (tissue homeostasis perspectives), 5-8
 for realignment (principles and guidelines), 12
 for recurrent patellar dislocation, 46-47
 for rotational malalignment (patella), 25

O

Ober's test, 46
Off label *vs.* on label chrondrocyte usage, 85
Osteochondral allografts, 95-97, 96f
Osteochondral autografts, 94-95, 95f
Osteochondral injuries, 39
Osteophytes (marginal and intralesional), 87
Osteotomy procedures, 26, 51, 62-63, 64, 68-69, 69f, 76-78, 77f
Outerbridge classification system, 86-87, 87f, 88t

P

Pain without malalignment (tissue homeostasis perspectives), 1-9
 ADLs, 5-6
 historical perspectives, 1, 1f-2f
 imaging techniques, 2-7
  MRI, 2-5
  Tc 99m-MDP scintigraphy, 2-7
 knee functions, 2-4, 4f
 patient histories, 5
 physical examinations, 5
 reference resources, 8-9
 tissue homeostasis theory, 1-2, 3t
 treatments, 5-8
  anti-inflammatory, 6

arthroscopic peripatellar synovectomy, 7-8, 7f
chondroplasty, 8
load restrictions, 6
McConnell taping, 6
nonsurgical, 5-7
painless muscle strengthening, 6
patellectomy, 8
patellofemoral taping, 6
realignment procedures (proximal and distal), 8
rehabilitation, 6-7
stretching, 6
surgical, 7-8, 7f
tissue cooling, 6
unicompartmental arthroplasty, 8
Painless muscle strengthening, 6
Patellar dislocation. *See also under individual topics*
 acute, 35-41
 recurrent, 43-55
Patellar hemiarthroplasty, 78-79, 78f
Patellectomy, 8, 80-81
Patellofemoral arthritis (isolated) without malalignment, 73-84. *See also* Isolated patellofemoral arthritis without malalignment
Patellofemoral arthroplasty, 78-79
Patellofemoral articular cartilage treatments, 85-99. *See also* Articular cartilage treatments
Patellofemoral chondrosis with associated tibiofemoral chondrosis, 88-89
Patellofemoral problems (common). *See also under individual topics*
 acute patellar dislocation, 35-41
 arthritis (patellofemoral) with malalignment, 57-71
 articular cartilage treatments, 85-99
 isolated patellofemoral arthritis without malalignment, 73-84
 mild patellar instability (arthroscopic reconstruction), 29-33
 pain without malalignment (tissue homeostasis perspectives), 1-9
 realignment (principles and guidelines), 11-17
 recurrent patellar dislocation, 43-55
 rotational malalignment (patella), 19-28
Patellofemoral realignment (principles and guidelines), 11-17. *See also* Realignment (principles and guidelines)
Patellofemoral taping, 6
Pathoanatomy-related issues, 29, 35-36, 35f-36f, 43, 47-48, 48t, 52
Pathology-related issues, 86, 86f
Pathomechanics, 45
Pathophysiology-related issues, 20, 20f
Patient histories. *See also under individual topics*
 for acute patellar dislocation, 39-40
 for arthritis (patellofemoral) with malalignment, 60
 for isolated patellofemoral arthritis without malalignment, 73-74
 for pain without malalignment (tissue homeostasis perspectives), 5
 for recurrent patellar dislocation, 44

for rotational malalignment (patella), 20
Patient selection criteria, 12
Physical examinations. *See also under individual topics*
 for acute patellar dislocation, 39-40
 for arthritis (patellofemoral) with malalignment, 60
 for isolated patellofemoral arthritis without malalignment, 73-74, 74*f*
 for pain without malalignment (tissue homeostasis perspectives), 5
 for recurrent patellar dislocation, 44-46
  lying prone, 45-46
  lying supine, 45
  side lying, 46
  sitting, 45
  standing, 44-45
  walking, 45
 for rotational malalignment (patella), 20-22, 21*f*-23*f*
Postoperative management, 51-52
Predisposition-related issues, 36-37
Procedure selection criteria, 59-60
Proximal realignment, 30-31, 31*f*
PTO Neoprene, 47

Q

Q angles, 22, 26, 30, 32-33, 45, 50, 58, 58*f*, 60-61, 63, 65*t*

R

Radiographs, 23-24, 24*f*, 32*f*, 36, 46, 57*f*, 58-60, 67*f*, 73, 73*f*, 77*f*, 80*f*, 86-87
Radionuclide imaging, 24
Realignment (principles and guidelines), 11-17
 associated problems, 11, 11*f*
 patient selection criteria, 12
 reference resources, 16-17
 treatments (nonsurgical), 12
 treatments (surgical), 12-16, 12*f*-15*f*
  arthroscopic medial imbrication, 13
  articular lesions and, 13
  complications, 16
  distal realignment, 14, 14*f*
  lateral release, 13, 13*f*
  medial patella resurfacing, 15
  MPFLs, 13-15, 14*f*
  soft-tissue pain sources and, 12-13, 12*f*
  tibial tubercle anteriorization and anteromedialization, 14-15, 14*f*-15*f*
  tissue quality assessments, 15-16
  trochleaplasty, 14
  VMO, 13
Reconstruction (arthroscopic), 29-33. *See also* Mild patellar instability (arthroscopic reconstruction)

Recurrent patellar dislocation, 43-55
 ACLs, 44
 biomechanics (patellar instability), 43-44
 epidemiology-related issues, 43
 imaging techniques, 43-52
  CT, 43, 46, 52
  MRI, 43, 46, 52
  radiographs, 46
 MPFLs, 43-44, 48-52
 natural history issues, 43
 pathoanatomy-related issues, 43, 47-48, 48*t*, 52
 patient histories, 44
 physical examinations, 44-46
  lying prone, 45-46
  lying supine, 45
  side lying, 46
  sitting, 45
  standing, 44-45
  walking, 45
 reference resources, 52-55
 treatments (nonsurgical), 46-47
 treatments (surgical), 46-52, 48*t*
  Albee osteotomy, 51
  historic, 46-47
  minimally invasive patellar realignment, 51
  outcomes, 46-47
  postoperative management, 51-52
  preferred, 47-52, 48*t*, 49*f*-51*f*
 VMO, 44-45, 47, 48*t*, 49-52
Reefing (medial), 30, 30*f*
Reference resources. *See also under individual topics*
 for acute patellar dislocation, 40-41
 for arthritis (patellofemoral) with malalignment, 69-71
 for articular cartilage treatments, 98-99
 for isolated patellofemoral arthritis without malalignment, 81-84
 for mild patellar instability (arthroscopic reconstruction), 33
 for pain without malalignment (tissue homeostasis perspectives), 8-9
 for realignment (principles and guidelines), 16-17
 for recurrent patellar dislocation, 52-55
 for rotational malalignment (patella), 26-28
Release (lateral), 13, 13*f*, 25, 30, 75-76
Retinacular release, 25
Rotational malalignment (patella), 19-28
 chondromalacia, 19-20
 differential diagnoses, 19, 19*f*
 imaging techniques, 22-26, 23*f*-24*f*
  CT, 22, 24, 26
  MRI, 22, 24, 26
  radiographs, 23-24, 24*f*
  radionuclide imaging, 24
pathophysiology-related issues, 20, 20*f*

patient histories, 20
physical examinations, 20-22, 21f-23f
    reference resources, 26-28
    treatments (nonsurgical), 25
        activity modifications, 25
        bracing, 25
        medication, 25
        physical therapy, 25
        shoe orthoses, 25
        taping, 25
    treatments (surgical), 25-26, 25f
        isolated lateral retinacular release, 25
        techniques, 25-26, 25f
        tibial tubercle transfers, 26

S

Scintigraphy (Tc 99m-MDP), 2-7
SF 36 (Medical Outcomes Study 36-Item Short Form Health
    Survey), 85
Shoe orthoses, 25
Side lying, 46
Sitting (physical examinations), 45
Soft-tissue pain sources, 12-13, 12f
Staining (Gomori trichrome), 20
Standing (physical examinations), 44-45
Static vs. dynamic factors (pathophysiology), 20
Stimulation (marrow), 92-93, 93f
Straight anteriorization, 69
Stretching, 6
Subluxation, 13, 13f, 30-31, 43, 45-46, 60-61, 63
Substance-P, 2
Surgical treatments. See also under individual topics
    for acute patellar dislocation, 38-39, 38t
    advantages, 29-33
    for isolated patellofemoral arthritis without malalignment,
        74-81
    for mild patellar instability (arthroscopic reconstruction),
        29-33
    for pain without malalignment (tissue homeostasis per-
        spectives), 5-8
    realignment (principles and guidelines), 12-16, 12f-15f
    for recurrent patellar dislocation, 46-52, 48t
    for rotational malalignment (patella), 25-26, 25f
Symptomatic arthrosis and anteromedialization, 63-69, 63t,
    64f, 65t, 66f-67f, 69f
Synovectomy, 7-8, 7f

T

Taping techniques, 6, 25
Technetium Tc 99m-MDP (methylene diphosphonate)
    scintigraphy, 2-7

Tibial tubercle anteriorization and anteromedialization, 14-15,
    14f-15f
Tibial tubercle elevation/osteotomy, 76-78, 77f
Tibiofemoral chondrosis, 88-89
Tilt-related issues, 13, 13f, 19-20, 19f, 60-61, 63, 73-74
Timing and balance (lower extremity), 11-12
Tinel's sign, 2
Tipping effect, 65t
Tissue cooling, 6
Tissue homeostasis perspectives, 1-9. See also Pain without
    malalignment (tissue homeostasis perspectives)
Tissue homeostasis theory, 1-2, 3t
Tissue quality assessments, 15-16
Torsional abnormalities, 57
Total knee arthroplasty, 80, 80f
Transfer (medial tibial tubercle), 60-63, 62f, 63t
Traumatic lesions, 90
Treatments. See also under individual topics
    nonsurgical
        for acute patellar dislocation, 37-38, 37t
        for isolated patellofemoral arthritis without malalignment,
            74
        for pain without malalignment (tissue homeostasis
            perspectives), 5-8
        for realignment (principles and guidelines), 12
        recurrent patellar dislocation, 46-47
        for rotational malalignment (patella), 25
    patient selection criteria, 12
    surgical
        for acute patellar dislocation, 38-39, 38t
        advantages, 29-33
        for arthritis (patellofemoral) with malalignment, 59-60
        for articular cartilage treatments, 91-97
        for isolated patellofemoral arthritis without malalignment,
            74-81
        for mild patellar instability (arthroscopic reconstruction),
            29-33
        for pain without malalignment (tissue homeostasis
            perspectives), 5-8
        postoperative management, 51-52
        procedure selection criteria, 59-60
        realignment (principles and guidelines), 12-16, 12f-15f
        for recurrent patellar dislocation, 46-52, 48t
        rotational malalignment (patella), 25-26, 25f
Trochleaplasty, 14
Trochlear dysplasia, 58
TruePull braces, 47
Tubercle malalignment, 57-59, 57f-59f

U

Unicompartmental arthroplasty, 8

V

Valgus alignment, 57
Vastus medialis obliquus (VMO), 13, 35-36, 35*f*-36*f*, 38-39
Venous congestion, 20
VMO (vastus medialis obliquus), 13, 35-36, 35*f*-36*f*, 38-39
Volumetric MRI (magnetic resonance imaging), 87

W

Walking (physical examinations), 45

Y

Yamamoto technique, 30

Keep informed on a broad range of topics with these Monographs

Four easy ways to order!

1. **PHONE** (credit card orders) AAOS toll-free **(800) 626-6726** Monday through Friday, 8:00 am to 5:00 pm, Central Time. Customers outside of the U.S. and Canada, call ++(847) 823-7186. **Please mention priority code 1870.**

2. **FAX** your purchase order and/or completed order form and credit card information toll-free to **(800) 823-8025**. Customers outside of the U.S. and Canada, fax to ++(847) 823-8025.

3. **ONLINE** (secure credit card orders) via the Academy's Home Page at **www.aaos.org.** Select "Educational Resources Catalog," then search by product or topic.

4. **MAIL** your completed order form with check to **AAOS, P.O. Box 75838, Chicago, Illinois 60675-5838** (please allow three to four weeks for delivery). Send credit card payment directly to **AAOS, 6300 N. River Road, Rosemont, Illinois 60018-4262.** Prices are subject to change without notice.

Shipping and Handling

Order Amount	U.S. (UPS Ground)
$35.01 to $75.00	**$7.95**
$75.01 to $100.00	**$9.95**
$100.01 to $200.00	**$13.95**
$200.01 or $250.00	**$16.95**
Over $250.00	**$19.95**
Canada residents add $10.00 surcharge to rates above	

☑ Yes! Send me the monographs I have indicated.

Item no.	Title	Price	AAOS Member Price	Resident Price	Quantity	Total
02-758	**NEW! Common Patellofemoral Problems** John P. Fulkerson, MD, Editor	$50	$40	$40		
02-713	**NEW! Neck Pain** Jeffrey Fischgrund, MD, Editor	$50	$40	$40		
02-714	**NEW! Adolescent Idiopathic Scoliosis** Peter Newton, MD, Editor	$50	$40	$40		
02-693	**NEW! Complications in Orthopaedics: Pediatric Upper Extremity Fractures** Charles Price, MD, Editor	$50	$40	$40		
02-692	**NEW! Complications in Orthopaedics: Tibial Shaft Fractures** William M. Ricci, MD, Editor	$50	$40	$40		
02-679	**Management of Thoracolumbar Fractures** Charles A. Reitman, MD, Editor	$50	$40	$40		
02-609	**Management of Osteoarthritis of the Knee** Freddie H. Fu, MD, and Bruce D. Browner, MD, Editors	$50	$40	$40		
02-579	**Revision Total Knee Arthroplasty** Leo A. Whiteside, MD, Editor	$50	$40	$40		
02-523	**Revision Total Hip Arthroplasty** Wayne G. Paprosky, MD, FACS, Editor	$50	$40	$40		
02-574	**Multiple Ligamentous Injuries of the Knee in the Athlete** Robert C. Schenck Jr., MD, Editor	$50	$40	$40		
02-413	**Arthroscopic Meniscal Repair** W. Dilworth Cannon Jr., MD, Editor	$50	$40	$40		
02-479	**Chronic Ankle Pain in the Athlete** Glenn B. Pfeffer, MD	$50	$40	$40		
02-245	**The Female Athlete** Carol Teitz, MD	$50	$40	$40		
02-570	**The Traumatized Foot** Bruce J. Sangeorzan, MD, Editor	$50	$40	$40		
02-322	**Disorders of the Great Toe** Robert S. Adelaar, MD	$50	$40	$40		
02-556	**Carpal Fracture-Dislocations** Thomas E. Trumble, MD, Editor	$50	$40	$40		
02-385	**Fractures of the Distal Radius** Harris Gelman, MD	$50	$40	$40		
02-509	**Total Shoulder Arthroplasty** Lynn A. Crosby, MD, Editor	$50	$40	$40		
02-347	**The Rotator Cuff: Current Concepts and Complex Problems** Joseph P. Iannotti, MD, PhD	$50	$40	$40		

International customers: Email AAOS Customer Service at **custserv@aaos.org** for ordering information, including where to obtain Academy products in your geographical area.

Subtotal	
Illinois purchasers add 9% sales tax	
Shipping and handling (see chart at left)	
Total	

Method of Payment

❑ Check or money order payable to AAOS enclosed (U.S. funds only)

❑ Purchase order enclosed (P.O.s will be accepted from institutions only)

❑ Visa ❑ MasterCard ❑ American Express

_____ _____
Card Number   Exp Date

_____
Signature

Ship to:

_____ _____
Name   Academy ID Number

_____
Address

_____ _____ _____
City   State/Province   Zip/Postal Code

_____ _____
Daytime Telephone   Fax Number

_____
Email

Stay current on clinical issues and challenges:
Subscribe to the Monograph Series today and **SAVE!**

❑ **Yes! I want to subscribe to the Monograph Series!**
Receive each new monograph <u>immediately upon publication</u> —about 5 per year— at a $5 discount from the list or member price.

2/05

Priority Code 1870